DATE DUE

DEMCO, INC. 38-2931

Chemical Exposures

Chemical Exposures

Low Levels and High Stakes

Nicholas A. Ashford &
Claudia S. Miller

VNR **Van Nostrand Reinhold**
_____ **New York**

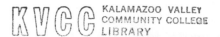

Library of Congress Catalog Number 90-38644
ISBN 0-442-00499-0

The research underlying this book was supported by the New
Jersey State Department of Health. Any opinions, findings,
conclusions, or recommendations expressed herein are those of
the authors and do not necessarily reflect the views of the New
Jersey State Department of Health, The Massachusetts Institute of
Technology, or The University of Texas.

Printed in the United States of America

Van Nostrand Reinhold
115 Fifth Avenue
New York, New York 10003

Chapman & Hall
2-6 Boundary Row
London SE1 8HN, England

Thomas Nelson Australia
102 Dodds Street
South Melbourne, Victoria 3205, Australia

Nelson Canada
1120 Birchmount Road
Scarborough, Ontario M1K 5G4, Canada

16 15 14 13 12 11 10 9 8 7 6 5 4 3 2

Library of Congress Cataloging-in-Publication Data

Ashford, Nicholas Askounes.
   Chemical exposures: low levels and high stakes/
Nicholas A. Ashford, Claudia S. Miller.
      p. cm.
   Includes bibliographical references and index.
   ISBN 0-442-00499-0
   1. Toxicology. 2. Pollution. 3. Environmental health.
I. Miller, Claudia, 1946–   . II. Title.
RA1216.A84   1991
363.17'91—dc20   90-38644
                                          CIP

To my mother, Venette Askounes Ashford, from whom I learned to have compassion for those less fortunate than I, and who inspired me to help.

—— N.A.A.

To my parents, Constance Lawrence Schultz and Ernst William Schultz, who patiently read stories to me as a child, encouraged my interest in science, and taught me to keep the two separated.

—— C.S.M.

Contents

Part II.
Mechanisms, Diagnosis, and Treatment / 85

Part III. Responding to the Problem / 145

Preface

Given the current controversies concerning the nature of chemical sensitivity and the fact that many physicians and scientists doubt that it is physical in origin, some words of explanation are in order for the readers of this book. At the beginning of the book, we describe patients who claim to be "chemically sensitive," that is, suffer acute adverse reactions to low levels of chemicals commonly found in homes, schools, places of employment, and other environments. In the ensuing pages, we drop the quotation marks and avoid terms such as "allegedly affected individuals" because their continual use would be awkward. Sufficient "proof" is not available to satisfy the most skeptical critic that chemical sensitivity exists as a physical entity, nor is there convincing proof that it does not. However, we are persuaded that the collective evidence, in part anecdotal and in part based on good scientific studies, does present a sufficiently compelling case to warrant further study. We cannot assert that millions of people are affected, although chemicals are ubiquitous and exposures are expected to continue. The size of the public health problem is unknown, but the scale of potential exposure suggests that the problem could be significant. We ask that readers approach this book with open minds and withhold judgment on these issues until they have read the entire book. A more focused second reading might also be needed.

Our purposes in undertaking the research underlying this book were: (1) to clarify the nature of chemical sensitivity and (2) to identify ways federal and state government can assist those who are affected. In undertaking this task, we reviewed much of the available scientific and medical literature relating to low-level chemical exposure and resulting disease. We also interviewed key individuals in various medical disciplines including allergy, clinical ecology, and occupational medicine. We found scientific and clinical evidence to support plausible hypotheses concerning this disorder. The evidence also offers fruitful areas for further research. In addition, we found areas of significant interprofessional conflict as well as areas of agreement. We noted an increasing desire by all parties to find a common ground from which the issues can be objectively and cooperatively addressed.

Much, but by no means all, anecdotal evidence for chemical sensitivities has been reported by clinical ecologists—physician practitioners whose clinical practices have come under intense criticism. However, chemical sensitivity is by no means the exclusive property of clinical ecology. The fields of occupational and environmental medicine contain sufficient examples to suggest a real medical problem. Our focus was on the problem of chemical sensitivity, not on the history of interprofessional conflict surrounding clinical ecology.

Some readers may be concerned that the lack of sufficient data in this area may render our conclusions speculative and hence biased. Certainly this book contains speculation. However, there is a difference between constructing rational hypotheses concerning the existence of chemical sensitivity based on all the evidence and engaging in unfounded conjecture. Finally, we hope that our efforts will stimulate others to undertake serious scientific inquiry into this fascinating and rapidly evolving area.

This book is divided into three parts. Part One defines the problem of chemical sensitivity. It discusses sensitive populations, low-level exposures to chemicals, the history of clinical ecology and its relationship to other disciplines, and the magnitude and nature of the problem. Part Two describes possible mechanisms, diagnostic approaches and therapies, and the areas of agreement and disagreement between allergists and clinical ecologists.

Part Three addresses research needs, patient and community concerns, health care, insurance, and compensation needs, the role of medical practitioners and their societies and recommendations for both research and action, given our present state of knowledge.

Acknowledgments

We are indebted to a number of people who gave generously of their time and energy to educate us on various issues and critique prior versions of the text. They include Iris Bell, Eddy Bresnitz, Mark Cullen, Linda Lee Davidoff, Nancy Fiedler, Ted Kniker, William Meggs, David Ozonoff, Theron Randolph, William Rea, Abba Terr, Lance Wallace, and Grace Ziem.

We are especially grateful to Kathleen Rest and Bob Miller, who both supported our effort and were our toughest critics. We thank Donald Beavers for research assistance on provocation-neutralization therapies.

In addition, we wish to thank the many people we contacted or interviewed in the course of our research. These people include Emil Bardana, Iris Bell, Eddy Bresnitz, Mark Cullen, Linda Lee Davidoff, Earon Davis, Kendall Gerdes, Bill Hirzy, Donald Jewett, Alfred Johnson, William King, William T. Kniker, Mary Lamielle, Alan Levin, William Meggs, Dean Metcalfe, Joseph Miller, David Ozonoff, Theron Randolph, Doris Rapp, William Rea, John Salvaggio, John Selner, Ray Slavin, John Spengler, Morton Teich, Abba Terr, Lance Wallace, Laura Welch, Grace Ziem, and many patients.

Finally, we thank Tom Burke of the New Jersey State Department of Health, for providing us the opportunity to investigate chemical sensitivity.

About the Authors

Nicholas A. Ashford, Ph.D., J.D., is Associate Professor of Technology and Policy at the Massachusetts Institute of Technology. He was Chairman of the National Advisory Committee on Occupational Safety and Health, served on the EPA Science Advisory Board, is a Fellow of the American Association for the Advancement of Science, and is currently Chairman of the Committee on Technology Innovation and Economics of the EPA National Advisory Council for Environmental Policy and Technology. He is the author of *Crisis in the Workplace: Occupational Disease and Injury* (1976), and co-author of *Evaluating Chemical Regulations: Trade-off Analysis and Impact Assessment for Environmental Decision-making* (1980), *Analyzing the Benefits of Health, Safety, and Environmental Regulations* (1982), *Monitoring the Worker for Exposure and Disease: Scientific and Ethical Considerations in the Use of Biomarkers* (1990), and *Technology, Law, and the Working Environment* (1991), Van Nostrand Reinhold. Dr. Ashford holds both a Doctorate in Chemistry and a Law Degree from the University of Chicago.

Claudia S. Miller, M.D., M.S., is Assistant Professor in Allergy and Immunology at the University of Texas Health Science Center at San Antonio, where she completed her fellowship in Allergy and Immunology. She is also board-certified in Internal Medicine and holds a Master's Degree in Environmental Health from the School of Public Health at the University of California at Berkeley. Dr. Miller served on the National Advisory Committee on Occupational Safety and Health. Before entering medicine, she was industrial hygienist for the University of California-San Francisco, OSHA's national training institute, and the United Steelworkers of America.

Introduction

Chemical exposures are endemic to our modern industrial society. Patients who believe they are chemically sensitive are caught up in an acrimonious cross fire among several different groups of physicians—traditional allergists; clinical ecologists; and in some cases, ear, nose and throat specialists; occupational physicians; and others. This acrimony is fueled by different medical paradigms of the definition, diagnosis, and treatment of disease or symptoms associated with exposure to low levels of chemicals in food and water, the outdoor environment, the work environment, indoor air, and consumer products. Legal conflicts further complicate the associated scientific and medical differences as attempts by "chemically sensitive" persons to obtain workers' compensation, disability payments, and damage awards from employers and from the producers and users of chemical products result in an adversary system that draws medical practitioners unwillingly into the center of the conflict. Further exacerbating the situation are the insurance industry and employers, who seek to reduce costs for medical care; their involvement continues the volatile history of economic tugs-of-war characteristic of health care in general. "Chemically sensitive" patients seek medical care and consideration from traditional medical practitioners, many of whom are ill equipped or reluctant to provide the painstaking and time-consuming attention that is required for this condition.

The research underlying this book was commissioned by the New Jersey State Department of Health in order to clarify the nature of chemical sensitivity and identify ways in which a state department of health can assist the chemically sensitive person and disengage the patient from the medical cross fire and its attendant conflicts. In this book we argue that both federal and state initiatives are needed. In undertaking this task, we reviewed much of the available scientific and medical literature relating to low-level chemical exposure and resulting disease. We interviewed key individuals in various medical disciplines including allergy, clinical ecology, and occupational medicine. This effort was facilitated by the fortuitous scheduling of national conferences by the allergists and by the clinical ecologists in the same 7-day period in Texas in February 1989. Physicians involved with the chemically sensitive patient are concerned about being drawn into a legal and political struggle that ultimately may not help the patient. Through our interviews we were able to identify not only areas of conflict between the allergists and clinical ecologists but also unexpected areas of common ground.

This book comes at a critical time. Since the government of Ontario completed a report on "environmental hypersensitivity disorders" (Thomson 1985) in 1985, sensitivity to chemicals has received unprecedented attention from many quarters in the United States. A "Workshop on Health Risks from Exposure to Common Indoor Household Products in Allergic or Chemically Diseased Persons" held by the National Academy of Sciences (NAS) on July 1, 1987, recommended an 18-month study to address the "15 percent of the U.S. population [who] have an increased allergic sensitivity to chemicals commonly found in household products, such as detergents, solvents, pesticides, metals and rubber, thus placing them at increased risk [of] disease" (National Research Council 1987). Although that study has not yet been funded, in 1989 the NAS convened a panel to examine the interrelationships of toxic exposures and immune response. Later the same year, the U.S. Office of Technology Assessment (OTA) began a study of noncancer risks of chemicals, including immunotoxicity. OTA completed a neurotoxicity study in 1990 [OTA 1990]. A Canadian national advisory committee held a work-shop on "environmental sensitivities" in May 1990 (Canada 1991). The NAS, in response to a request from the EPA's office of Indoor Air, conducted a multiple chemical sensitivity workshop in early 1991 to develop research protocols for the syndrome (Hileman 1991; National Research Council 1991).

The U.S. Congressional Research Service has issued a report on indoor air pollution in which chemical sensitivity is explicitly recognized (Courpas 1988, p. CRS-9). The Environmental Protection Agency (EPA) acknowledges that health problems exist with low-level exposures well below those allowed by existing regulations (Claussen 1988); in its *Report to Congress on Indoor Air Quality,* EPA identifies multiple chemical sensitivities as a health concern (EPA 1989, p. 16). The Superfund Amendments, SARA, Title IV mandate a vigorous investigation of the problems of indoor air pollution by EPA. John D. Spengler of Harvard's School of Public Health, a leading authority on indoor air pollution, has testified (1988):

> There is growing evidence that there are chemically sensitive individuals in our society. Many, it is believed, may have acquired the sensitivity due to chronic exposures. But even without frank illness, the syndrome of irritation, fatigue, shortness of breath and nausea associated with building-related problems results in lost productivity and wasteful investigations and litigation.

Legislation introduced in Congress (S.1629, H.R. 5373) explicitly recognizes multiple chemical sensitivities resulting from indoor air pollutants as a serious threat to public health. Maryland has completed a study of "chemical hypersensitivity syndrome" (Bascom 1989). Legislation establishing a demonstration program to provide services and assistance to chemically hypersensitive persons (S.696) is likely to be introduced in New Jersey. These activities underscore a ground swell of activity that requires in-depth and thoughtful attention to chemical sensitivity.

We are at a critical crossroads. We have at this time a small window of opportunity that may close if we do not take action to address the problems of the chemically sensitive individual in a caring and equitable way. The recommendations in this book result from our interviews, literature review, and examination of the issues, and we suggest that their adoption is necessary for making substantial progress in this area. As the second printing of this book goes to press, both a Canadian national advisory committee (Canada 1991) and The U.S. National Research Council (National Research Council 1991) have formulated specific recommendations that have the potential to take the issue of chemical sensitivity into mainstream medicine and public health.

PART · I

Defining Chemical Sensitivity

CHAPTER 1

Chemical Exposures and Sensitive Populations

Groups Sensitive to Low-level Chemical Exposure

A review of the literature on exposure to low levels of chemicals reveals four groups or clusters of people with heightened reactivity:

1. Industrial workers
2. Occupants of "tight buildings," including office workers and school-children
3. Residents of communities whose air or water is contaminated by chemicals
4. Individuals who have had personal and unique exposures to various chemicals in domestic indoor air, pesticides, drugs, and consumer products

These four groups are listed for comparison in Table 1-1. Note that they differ in professional and educational attainment, age and sex, and the mix and levels of chemicals to which they are exposed, but that all have multiple symptoms involving multiple organ systems with marked variability in the type and degree of those symptoms. Symptoms are often "subjective." For example, central nervous system (CNS) symptoms such

TABLE 1-1. Chemically Sensitive Groups

Group	Nature of Exposure	Demographics
Industrial workers	Acute and chronic exposure to industrial chemicals	Primarily males; blue collar; 20 to 65 years old
Tight-building occupants	Off-gassing from construction materials, office equipment or supplies; tobacco smoke; inadequate ventilation	Females more than males; white-collar office workers and professionals; 20 to 65 years old; schoolchildren
Contaminated communities	Toxic waste sites, aerial pesticide spraying, ground water contamination, air contamination by nearby industry and other community exposures	All ages, male and female; children or infants may be affected first or most; pregnant women with possible effects on fetuses; middle to lower class
Individuals	Heterogeneous; indoor air (domestic), consumer products, drugs, and pesticides	70–80% females; 50% 30 to 50 years old (Johnson and Rea 1989); white, middle to upper middle class and professionals

as difficulty concentrating or irritability are common, and physical examinations are frequently unremarkable for individuals in each category. Careful analysis of these groups may reveal differences that can illuminate the etiologies and suggest effective therapeutic options for the myriad problems comprising chemical sensitivity. These differences also may create a referral or selection bias such that members of the four groups present themselves preferentially to different medical practitioners; some may consult occupational health physicians, others primary care physicians, and still others clinical ecologists or allergists (see Chapter 6).

Problems experienced by people in tight buildings, by industrial workers in a particular workplace, or by the residents of a contaminated community often occur within a relatively short time period—perhaps weeks or a few months. These problems may occur after a recognized event such as the installation of new carpeting, relocation to a new workplace, or changes in workplace or community exposures. The temporal cohesiveness of exposures and problems can contribute to the recognition of the problem as real. Acceptance of these problems as bona fide physical disease may also be facilitated by the recognition that these problems are widespread in nature and simply are not limited to what some observers would describe as malingering employees, hysterical housewives, and workers experiencing mass psychogenic illness. We are struck by the fact that individuals in such demographically divergent groups as those in Table 1-1, including industrial workers, office workers, housewives, and children, report similar polysymptomatic complaints triggered by chemical exposures. Perhaps some common thread unites these individuals. The similarities of both their medical complaints and their exposure histories may be more than coincidental.

In a survey of some 6,800 persons claiming to be chemically sensitive, 80 percent asserted they knew "when, where, with what, and how they were made ill" (National Foundation for the Chemically Hypersensitive 1989). Of the 80 percent, 60 percent (that is, almost half of those who replied) blamed pesticides. The respondents to the survey were self selected, and the results must be interpreted with caution. Nevertheless, the results indicate that future surveys of persons with different exposure histories and symptoms might contribute to an understanding of underlying mechanisms and causes.

In some chemically sensitive patients, no single, identifiable, "high-level" exposure seems to have been associated with the onset of their difficulties. Exposures may have occurred but were not recognized or remembered. Some observers suggest that repetitive or cumulative lower-level exposure events may lead to the development of sensitivities. Still others implicate genetic predisposition, pregnancy, major surgery with anesthesia, physical trauma, or major psychological stress as contributors to the illness (see Chapter 4).

Types of Sensitivity

The different meanings of the term *sensitivity* are at least partially responsible for the confusion surrounding chemical sensitivity.

Individuals differ in their responses to increasing doses of a toxic substance. The underlying causes of interindividual variability include age, sex, and genetic makeup; lifestyle and behavioral factors, including nutritional and dietary factors; alcohol, tobacco, and drug use; environmental factors; and preexisting disease (Ashford et al. 1984). In the classical, toxicological use of the word *sensitivity*, those individuals who require relatively lower doses to induce a particular response are said to be more sensitive than those who would require relatively higher doses before experiencing the same response (Hattis et al. 1987). A hypothetical distribution of sensitivities, that is, the minimum doses necessary to cause individuals in a population to exhibit a harmful effect, is shown in curve *A* in Figure 1-1. (If we plot the cumulative number of individuals who exhibit a particular response as a function of dose, we generate a population dose-response curve; see curve *A* in Figure 1-2.) This distribution describes the traditional toxicological concept of sensitivity. Curve *A* in Figure 1-1 illustrates that health effects of classical diseases

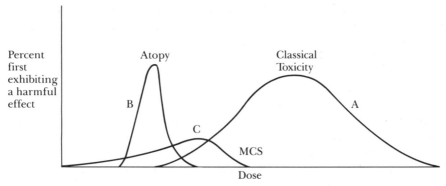

FIGURE 1-1.   *Hypothetical distribution of different types of sensitivities as a function of dose. Curve A is a sensitivity distribution for classical toxicity, e.g., to lead or a solvent. Sensitive individuals are found in the left-hand tail of the distribution. Curve B is a sensitivity distribution of atopic or allergic individuals in the population who are sensitive to an allergen, e.g., ragweed or bee venom. Curve C is a sensitivity distribution for individuals with multiple chemical sensitivities who, because they are already sensitized, subsequently respond to particular incitants, e.g., formaldehyde or phenol.*

are seen in a significant portion of the normal population at a certain dose; the sensitive and resilient populations are found in the tails of the distribution. (Of course, not all toxic substances have large variances or significant tails.) Painstaking scientific research and removing the effects of confounding variables have resulted in the discovery of sensitive individuals at levels heretofore considered safe. Recent work on lead (Bellinger et al. 1987) and benzene (Rinsky et al. 1987) are just two examples. For the sensitive person, avoidance of low-level exposures generally leads to improvement, or at least to the arrest of the development of the disease.

A second meaning of the word *sensitivity* appears in the context of classical IgE-mediated allergy (atopy). IgE is one of five classes of antibodies made by the body, and is, from the perspective of classically allergic individuals, the most important antibody. Atopic individuals have IgE directed against specific environmental incitants, such as ragweed or bee venom. Positive skin tests in these individuals correlate with a rapid onset of symptoms when they are actually exposed to those allergens. The atopic individual exhibits a reaction whereas nonallergic persons do not, even at the highest doses normally found in the environment. A hypothetical sensitivity distribution for an atopic effect is shown in curve *B* of Figure 1-1, and the dose-response curve derived from that distribution is found in curve *B* of Figure 1-2.

Allergists include in the term *allergy* well-characterized immune responses that result from industrial exposure to certain chemicals, such

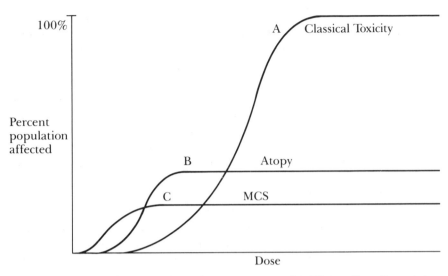

FIGURE 1-2. Hypothetical population dose-response curves for different effects. Curve A is a cumulative dose-response curve for classical toxicity, e.g., to lead or a solvent. Curve B is a cumulative dose-response curve for atopic or allergic individuals in the population who are sensitive to an allergen, e.g., ragweed or bee venom. Curve C is a cumulative dose-response curve for individuals with multiple chemical sensitivities who, because they are already sensitized, subsequently respond to particular incitants, e.g., formaldehyde or phenol.

as nickel or toluene diisocyanate (TDI). Most allergists refer to such responses as *chemical sensitivity,* and reserve this term for responses that have a distinct immunological basis, preferring to use a term such as *chemical intolerance* for nonimmunological responses to chemicals.

Patients suffering from multiple chemical sensitivities may be exhibiting a third and entirely different type of sensitivity. Their health problems often (but not always) appear to originate with some acute or traumatic exposure, after which the triggering of symptoms and observed sensitivities occur at very low levels of chemical exposure. The inducing chemical or substance may or may not be the same as the substances that thereafter provoke or "trigger" responses. (Sometimes the inducing substance is described as "sensitizing" the individual and the affected person as a "sensitized" person.) Reactions may sometimes be observed at incitant levels similar to those to which classically sensitive and atopic patients respond. Unlike classical toxicity, however, here the effects of low-level exposures are not simply those effects observed in normal populations at higher doses. The fact that normal persons—for example, most doctors—do not experience even at *higher* levels of exposure those symptoms that chemically sensitive patients describe at much lower levels of exposure probably helps to explain the reluctance of some physicians to believe that the problems are physical in nature. (Although this also describes atopy, here the sensitivity is not IgE mediated.) To compound the problem of physician acceptance of this illness, multiple organ systems may be affected, and multiple substances may trigger the effects. Over time, sensitivities seem to spread, in terms of both the types of triggering substances and the systems affected (Randolph 1962, pp. 98 and 119). Avoidance of the offending substances is usually effective but much more difficult to achieve for these patients than for classically sensitive patients because symptoms may occur at extremely low doses and the exposures are ubiquitous. Adaptation to chronic low-level exposure with consequent "masking" of symptoms (discussed more fully later) may make it exceedingly difficult to discover these sensitivities and unravel the multifactorial triggering of symptoms. A hypothetical sensitivity distribution for a single symptom for the already chemically sensitive person in response to a single substance trigger is shown in curve *C* of Figure 1-1, and the corresponding dose-response curve is shown in curve *C* of Figure 1-2. It should be emphasized, however, that individuals who become chemically sensitive may have been exposed to an initial *priming* event that was *toxic*, as classically defined.

Conceivably, exposure to certain substances, such as formaldehyde, might elicit all three types of sensitivities.

The fact that sensitivity means something quite different to toxicologists, allergists, and clinical ecologists reflects the different disease paradigms under which each operates. Neither traditional allergists nor toxicologists fully appreciate the two-step process of induction and triggering that seems to characterize multiple chemical sensitivities.

Those clinical ecologists who reference the literature on classical chemical toxicity to buttress their case for chemical sensitivity may be adding to the confusion and contributing to others' reluctance to accept their ideas. Likewise, allergists who dismiss chemical sensitivity on the grounds that it is not consistent with a recognized immunologic mechanism may be overlooking another kind of sensitivity in their patients. Although chemicals may act in some manner (via a toxic mechanism, for instance), to predispose or cause the body to be reactive to subsequent low-level chemical exposures, the *resulting* hyperreactivity to low levels of chemically diverse and unrelated substances is not toxicity as classically defined or understood at this time (see Chapter 4). Some allergists maintain that the term *chemical sensitivity* should not be used in the context we have used here, but should be reserved only for those responses having an immunological basis. We feel that the term *sensitivity* has broader applicability. A parallel might be the word *resistance*, which is widely understood whether one is talking about electricity, psychiatry, or an infectious disease. Similarly, *sensitivity* is easily understood when used in any of the three contexts illustrated in this section; it is not the exclusive property of the atopist.

Cullen (1987a) proposes that individuals with well-defined clinical entities such as asthma should not be given a diagnosis of multiple chemical sensitivities. Yet asthma may be one of the manifestations of this syndrome. It is important not to confuse diagnosis with etiology. The extent to which occupational asthma may overlap with multiple chemical sensitivity needs study and clarification. Classically, asthma has been divided into two categories: *extrinsic* asthma triggered by allergic (IgE) responses to pollens, dust, mold, and so on, and *intrinsic* asthma in which exposures outside the individual are not felt to play a causative role. The etiology of intrinsic asthma is ill-defined. Physicians have long warned their asthmatic patients to avoid irritants such as cigarette smoke, perfume, and strong cleaning agents, suggesting that such exposures might further irritate vulnerable airways, making their asthma worse. Few physicians, however, would view these irritants as a primary cause of their patients' asthma. Yet chronic irritation of any kind can lead to inflammation. Increasingly, the pathogenesis of asthma is being recognized as inflammation of the airways, and the most effective therapies for asthma are considered to be anti-inflammatory drugs such as cromolyn or steroids. Thus, asthma *is* inflammation, and inflammation can be caused by irritants, chemical or otherwise. Hence, it is quite possible that some asthma formerly designated as *intrinsic* may turn out to be external or *extrinsic* in origin, when the pathways leading to inflammation are delineated. Indeed, some feel that recent upward trends in asthma morbidity and mortality parallel increases in atmospheric pollution. Recently, a new clinical entity called reactive airway dysfunction syndrome (RADS) which shares certain features of multiple chemical sensitivity (Brooks 1985), has been described. Like multiple chemical sensitivity, RADS may be triggered by a single massive chemical exposure, for example, a chemical spill or fire. Subsequently, low levels of many common chemicals, (e.g., cigarette smoke, detergents, or perfume) that had never caused problems before may trigger airway constriction.

Physicians who see more or less random individuals who are not members of an identifiable exposure group are less likely to recognize patterns or similarities among these patients who claim to be chemically sensitive. Now that more attention is being focused on problems of industrial workers, occupants of tight buildings, and families in contaminated communities, these "random" patients (the fourth group in Table 1-1) may be diagnosed more readily. Once physicians recognize a constellation of symptoms that occurs repeatedly in individuals who share similar exposure histories, the disease seems to change its label from "idiopathic" or "psychogenic" to a recognized disorder, such as has occurred in the case of sick building syndrome (Kreiss 1989). Cullen's recent book (1987) on multiple chemical sensitivities was stimulated by his observations of a particular pattern of symptoms among workers which was previously unfamiliar to most occupational physicians. In the future, patterns observed in occupational and other cohesive groups of patients should facilitate a better understanding of what seems to many to be a hopeless confusion of reported symptoms.

Changes in Chemical Production and Use, and the Emergence of Chemical Sensitivity

In the conclusion to his *Workers with Multiple Chemical Sensitivities,* Cullen (1987b, p. 804) writes:

> The health problems of workers who react to low levels of environmental pollutants and chemicals, increasingly reported and recognized in recent years, has [*sic*] posed a serious dilemma for health providers from a wide array of disciplines, including generalists, internists, family practitioners, allergists, psychiatrists, social workers, and frequently occupational physicians and nurses. The inability of these professionals to provide satisfactory care from the patient's perspective has led to the emergence of new and alternative clinical theories and approaches, challenging traditional views. Unfortunately, the success of these alternative approaches has also not been demonstrated, fueling an ever widening and hostile debate in which *the patient is held hostage and virtually all clinicians are rendered impotent because of widely known intraprofessional disagreements.* [emphasis added]

How did these disagreements arise? Why are more and more problems related to low-level exposure to chemicals being reported in recent years? Is the problem merely increasingly recognized, or are the numbers of individuals being affected actually increasing? We shall try to shed some light on these questions by examining the development of this problem and the changes in chemical production, consumer products, and building design that have accompanied its emergence. We also include a brief history of clinical ecology, noting its split from allergy, subsequent growth, and continued conflicts with traditional allergists.

The increased medical interest in exposure to chemicals, especially low-level exposures, accompanied changes in the production of synthetic organic chemicals, building construction, and indoor air quality.

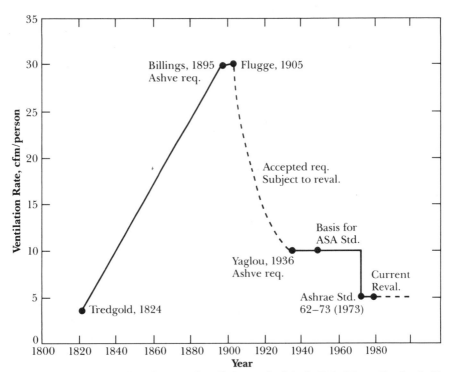

FIGURE 1-3. *Historical development of ventilation standards in the United States. Reprinted with permission from Mage, D. and R. Gammage, "Evaluation of Changes in Outdoor Air Quality Occurring Over the Past Several Decades," in* Indoor Air and Human Health, *R. Gammage and S. Kaye, Eds. (copyright 1985, Lewis Publishers, Inc., Chelsea, MI) p. 13.*

With the concern for energy conservation in the 1970s, homes and office buildings in the United States were constructed more tightly and make-up air (fresh air intake) was cut to a minimum. The historical trend of ventilation standards, used by architects and building designers, can be seen in Figure 1-3. The earliest standard, proposed by Tredgold in 1824 to prevent stuffiness, provided 4 cubic feet per minute (cfm) fresh make-up air per occupant. In 1893 Billings recommended 30 cfm per person, a value subsequently adopted by the American Society of Heating and Ventilation Engineers (ASHVE) and incorporated into the building codes of 22 states by 1925. In 1936 this standard was lowered to 10 cfm per person in response to research by Yaglou on the threshold of detection for human body odors; the American Standards Association adopted this value in 1946. Thus, before the energy crisis of 1973, odor detection was the basis for the ventilation standard. In the mid-1970s, as a result of energy concerns, ASHRAE (American Society of Heating,

Refrigeration and Air Conditioning Engineers) lowered the standard to 5 cfm per occupant, and 45 states adopted this standard into their codes in disregard of studies indicating that more fresh air was needed to dilute human odors and tobacco smoke to comfortable levels (Morey and Shattuck 1989). In 1981 ASHRAE revised the standard to 20 cfm of fresh air per occupant in areas where smoking is allowed. The current standard, issued in 1989, recommends at least 15 cfm per person, regardless of smoking. Fifteen cfm per person in schools, 20 cfm in offices, and 25 cfm in hospital rooms are recommended, with even higher rates if air from the ventilation system does not adequately mix with room air breathed by occupants or if unusual sources of contaminants are present (Morey and Shattuck 1989). However, from the mid-1970s into the 1980s, many commercial buildings were designed in accordance with the 5-cfm-per-occupant ASHRAE standard.

Similarly, beginning in the 1970s homeowners and new home builders caulked and sealed, installed storm windows and extra insulation, and effectively reduced fresh air infiltration. Homes, unlike commercial buildings, do not have ventilation systems that supply fresh make-up air, but rely on infiltration through doors, windows, cracks, and crevices instead. Such repairs were economically advantageous and in part tax deductible. In older homes not given these energy overhauls, the average fresh air infiltration rate is almost twice that of newer homes (0.9 versus 0.5 air changes per hour), but individual homes vary tremendously from 0.1 to more than 3 air changes per hour (Mage and Gammage 1985). See Figure 1-4.

More than 800 different volatile compounds were observed inside four buildings studied by the EPA (Wallace 1985). Wallace summarizes recent studies of indoor air pollutants:

1. Indoor median concentrations of volatile organics are consistently greater, by factors of 2 to 5, than outdoor medians.

2. At higher concentrations, the indoor-outdoor ratio increases, often beyond factors of 10.

3. Concentrations are extremely variable, covering 3 to 4 orders of magnitude, indicating the presence of intense indoor sources.

4. These sources are many, including paints, adhesives, cleansers, cosmetics, and other consumer products and building materials; but also common activities, such as visiting the dry cleaner shop or even taking a hot shower!

EPA conducted TEAM (Total Exposure Assessment Methodology) studies on a variety of volatile organics (1980–1987), carbon monoxide (1982–1983), pesticides (1986–1989), and particulates (1987–present).

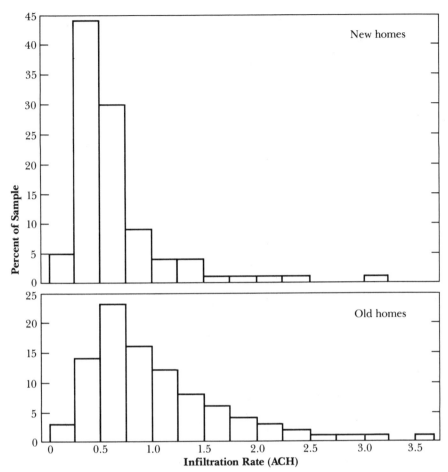

FIGURE 1-4. *Infiltration rates in U.S. houses in air changes per hour (ACH). Reprinted with permission from Mage, D. and R. Gammage, "Evaluation of Changes in Outdoor Air Quality Occurring Over the Past Several Decades, in* Indoor Air and Human Health, *R. Gammage and S. Kaye, Eds. (copyright 1985, Lewis Publishers, Inc., Chelsea, MI), p. 16.*

The goals of the studies were to develop methods for measuring individual total exposure and resulting body burden of toxic and carcinogenic organic chemicals and to estimate the exposures and body burdens of urban populations in several U.S. cities. Representative data from a study of 20 volatile organic compounds in the personal (indoor) air, outdoor air, drinking water, and breath of approximately 400 residents of New Jersey, North Carolina, and North Dakota are shown in Figures 1-5 and 1-6 (Wallace 1987).

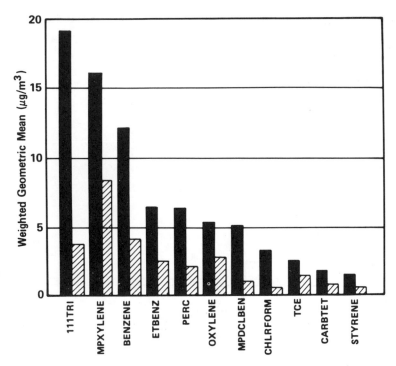

FIGURE 1-5.   Comparison of indoor and outdoor exposures to toxic compounds. Estimated geometric means of 11 toxic compounds in overnight (6:00 PM to 6:00 AM) air samples for the target population (128,000) of Elizabeth and Bayonne, New Jersey, between September and November 1981. Personal air (i.e., indoor) estimates (solid) are based on 347 samples and outdoor air estimates (hatched) are based on 84 samples. Compound abbreviations are: 1,1,1TRI, 1,1,1-trichloroethane; MPXYLENE, m,p-xylene; ETBENZ, ethylbenzene; PERC, tetrachloroethylene; OXYLENE, o-xylene; MPDCLBEN, m,p-dichlorobenzene; CHLRFORM, chloroform; TCE, trichloroethylene; CARBTET, carbon tetrachloride.
Source: Wallace, L. et al., "The TEAM Study: Personal Exposures to Toxic Substances in Air, Drinking Water, and Breath of 400 Residents of New Jersey, North Carolina, and North Dakota," Environmental Research (1987) 43:290–307, Academic Press, San Diego, California, p. 297.

Ten of the 11 chemicals measured in the breath of New Jersey residents correlated significantly with indoor air exposure levels, which were uniformly higher than outdoor levels (Fig. 1-5). Only for chloroform did breath levels correlate more closely with drinking water concentrations. Breath levels for most chemicals measured were 30–40 percent of indoor air levels, but measured up to 90 percent of indoor air levels in some cases—tetrachloroethylene, for example. A study of non-occupational pesticide exposure (Fig. 1-7) also shows dramatically higher concentrations of pesticides indoors than out of doors [Immerman 1990].

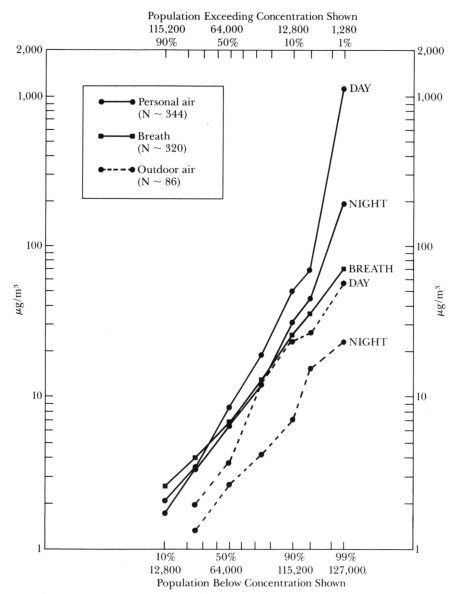

FIGURE 1-6. *Tetrachloroethylene in indoor air, outdoor air and breath. Estimated frequency distributions of tetrachloroethylene in personal air exposures, outdoor air concentrations, and exhaled breath values for the combined Elizabeth-Bayonne target population (128,000). All air values are 12-hr integrated samples. The breath value was taken following the daytime air sample (6:00 AM–6:00 PM). All outdoor air samples were taken in the vicinity of the participants' homes.*
Source: *Wallace, L., et al., "The TEAM Study: Personal Exposures to Toxic Substances in Air, Drinking Water, and Breath of 400 Residents of New Jersey, North Carolina, and North Dakota,* Environmental Research *(1987) 43:290–307. Academic Press, San Diego, California, p. 296.*

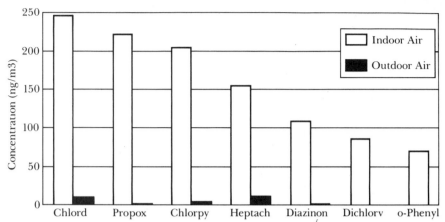

FIGURE 1-7. *Pesticide concentrations in indoor and outdoor air (Jacksonville, FL).*
Source: *Immerman 1990.*

Remarkably, these sources present in indoor air are the same ones individuals with multiple chemical sensitivities identify as provoking their vague and seemingly inexplicable symptoms. With their homes and workplaces already filled with synthetic materials that off-gas, gas furnaces, cigarette smoke, and other sources of pollutants, Americans sealed their buildings for energy efficiency. Not surprisingly, indoor air pollution levels rose dramatically, and so did health complaints. In addition, Americans spend many more hours per day indoors at work and at home, in schools, shopping malls, and other buildings than preceding generations (Environmental Protection Agency 1989, Massachusetts 1989).

With indoor air pollution on the rise since World War II and tighter, more energy-efficient construction of schools and workplaces, outbreaks of sick building syndrome appeared in the late 1970s. Chlorine production is felt by some to provide a useful index of the increased quantities of synthetic organics that are found indoors (e.g., polyvinyl chloride). Figure 1-8 shows the dramatic rise in chlorine production in billions of pounds per year that has occurred since World War II, plotted against mean sperm density, a widely recognized and subtle indicator of the toxic effects of a variety of chemicals, for example, lead. Actually, increases in chlorine production underestimate increases in the amount of synthetic organics. Figure 1-9 depicts production changes since 1945. Before World War II, U.S. production of synthetic organic chemicals totaled fewer than a billion pounds per year. By 1976, production had soared to 163 billion pounds annually (Odell 1980, p. 213). Increased sources of indoor air pollution, coupled with decreased fresh make-up

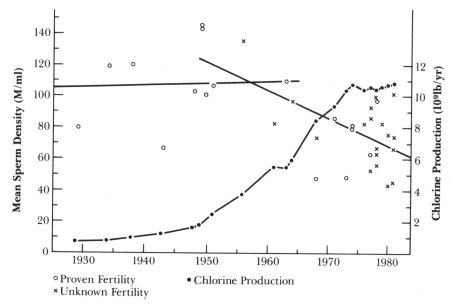

FIGURE 1-8. *Increasing chlorine production in the U.S. and the apparent reduction in human sperm density. Reprinted with permission from Mage, D. and R. Gammage, "Evaluation of changes in Outdoor Air Quality Occurring Over the Past Several Decades," in* Indoor Air and Human Health, *R. Gammage and S. Kaye, Eds. (copyright 1985, Lewis Publishers, Inc., Chelsea, MI) p. 10.*

air, have transformed the indoor environment. Community exposures to toxic chemicals, industrial and office exposures, and other episodic exposures of individuals also increased, reflecting the rise in production of coal- and oil-derived chemicals and synthetics.

These changes in chemical production, consumer products, and building design have been accompanied by an increasing number of people who appear to react to low levels of environmental pollutants. Indeed, since World War II certain illnesses, such as asthma (Sly 1988) and depression (Klerman and Weissman 1989), seem to have shown upsurges. Many patients with these conditions and other health problems, frustrated by their lack of success with traditional medicine, sought the care of clinical ecologists, who related their patients' symptoms to environmental exposures.

Theron Randolph, who founded clinical ecology, and a number of other clinical ecologists are board-certified allergists. Randolph received his M.D. degree from the University of Michigan, where he completed his residency in internal medicine. His allergy and immunology fellowship was completed at Massachusetts General Hospital and Harvard

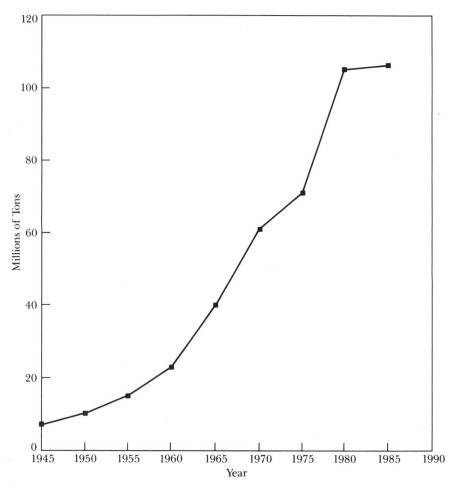

FIGURE 1-9.   *Synthetic organic chemical production United States, 1945–1985.*
Source: U.S. Intern. Trade Commission.

Medical School in 1942 to 1944. He entered private practice in Chicago, where he also served as a clinical instructor in allergy at Northwestern University Medical School for several years. Randolph reported that many of his patients reacted adversely to common foods such as corn (a food ubiquitous in the American diet in the form of sugar, starch, and oil, as well as in its unrefined state), wheat, milk, and eggs. Indeed, he later described corn allergy as "the most common food allergy in North America" (Randolph and Moss 1980, p. 109). He used Rinkel's technique (Rinkel 1944; Rinkel et al. 1951) of having patients avoid specific foods for 4 to 6 days (and not much longer) to "unmask" reactions prior to test-feeding them. Herbert Rinkel, another American allergist, had first described the phenomenon of "masking" and its clinical application for food sensitivities.

According to ecologists, most allergists then, as now, do not recognize or employ this avoidance or "unmasking" period prior to testing and thus never see this type of food sensitivity in their patients. Recent guidelines on food testing written for allergists and published in their journal do not address this issue (Bock et al. 1988). Many traditional allergists recognize primarily IgE-mediated, immediate reactions to foods that generally are more readily observable by the investigator and do not require an avoidance period in order to detect them.

In 1951, Randolph realized that not only foods but also chemicals might be responsible for some of his patients' symptoms. A physician's wife who sold cosmetics had been seeing Randolph over a 4-year period for rhinitis, asthma, headache, fatigue, irritability, depression, markedly fluctuating weight, and intermittent episodic loss of consciousness (Randolph 1987, pp. 73–76). At each visit, he recorded almost verbatim on his typewriter the patient's statements about her condition, without editing. By 1951, he had compiled 50 single-spaced typewritten pages concerning this woman. Reading over these pages, he realized there was a common denominator: each event was associated with exposure to gas, oil, coal, or their combustion products. Similar observations in other patients followed. A few years later, Randolph published a series of six abstracts in the *Journal of Laboratory and Clinical Medicine* concerning "allergic type" reactions to industrial solvents and liquid fuels, mosquito abatement fogs and mists, motor exhausts, indoor utility gas and oil fumes, and chemical (coal or petrochemically derived) additives in foods, drugs, and cosmetics (Randolph 1954 a–f).

Randolph and other ecologists often refer to chemical sensitivities as the "petrochemical problem" because the increase in the incidence of this illness seems to parallel the growth of the petrochemical industry and the increased use of synthetic materials such as particleboard, pesticides, synthetic textiles, plastics, and food additives by consumers since World War II. Late in the 1950s, Randolph adopted the term *clinical ecology* in order to describe his practice and its focus on environmental incitants and in order to avoid use of the word *allergy*.

Randolph, who had been hospitalizing patients and testing them for their food sensitivities, found that another critical element in many of his patients' recoveries was avoidance of environmental chemical exposures in their jobs and/or homes while in the hospital. He developed "Comprehensive Environmental Control," a diagnostic approach in which patients avoid exposure to synthetic chemicals in order to facilitate diagnosis of chemical sensitivity. The next chapter describes this method in detail. A description of comprehensive environmental control and its role in diagnosis and therapy first appeared 30 years ago in *Clinical Physiology* (Randolph 1960) and again in the *Annals of Allergy* in 1965 (Randolph 1965); *Human Ecology and Susceptibility to the Chemical Environment* lists the most common chemical exposures Randolph felt provoked symptoms in his patients (Randolph 1962).

Although Randolph reported treating a wide range of illnesses successfully, his and other clinical ecologists' enthusiasm for this approach was not shared by many of their contemporaries. Randolph's early work showing that environmental influences can provoke mental and behavioral disturbances in a demonstrable, cause-and-effect way occurred in the 1950s, at the same time modern psychopharmacology was developing and the use of phenothiazine tranquilizers was expanding. Drugs that could control behavior, so-called chemical restraints, were easy to administer and mass applicable, and drug companies promoted them widely. University research in psychiatry, funded by drug companies, became focused on the development of better drugs. Only later were the long-range complications of many of these drugs realized. The dominance of psychoanalytical, behavioral, and pharmacological approaches to mental illness abrogated any major attempts by psychiatrists to look for food or chemical triggers for their patients' illnesses (Randolph 1987, p. 188). Randolph and other clinical ecologists are critical of these developments in psychiatry: "especially psychoanalysis, despite its wide application, has been devoid of any demonstrable evidence of etiology and has been relatively ineffective therapeutically" (Randolph 1987, pp. 190–191).

As clinical ecologists continued to apply their concepts of environmental illness, many of which did *not* appear dependent upon immune mechanisms, they distanced themselves more and more from traditional allergists. When von Pirquet coined the name *allergy* in 1906, he defined it as "altered reactivity" of whatever origin. Thus the word *allergy* as originally used embraced both immunity and hypersensitivity (Corwin 1985). In 1925 European allergists influenced their American colleagues to redefine *allergy* in the context of antibodies and antigens. Randolph, Coca, and other allergists objected, preferring to call this development the "immunologic theory of allergy," but the new definition prevailed. Thus clinical ecology, which was concerned with heightened reactivity of unknown etiology, did not fit under this new definition. In 1967, when IgE was discovered, it enhanced allergy's credibility as a specialty. (At the time, allergy shots were dimly viewed, even called "witchcraft" or "voodoo medicine" by some medical practitioners.) IgE's discovery provided allergists with a scientific basis for their practice, and some began to look down on areas such as clinical ecology that did not have such a basis. Thus the observations of clinical ecologists, irrespective of their validity or clinical utility, were excluded from allergy, in part because IgE did not appear to be involved. Allergy and clinical ecology have continued to develop and define their separate paradigms. Tables 1-2 and 1-3 present the salient differences in approach and philosophy.

These dueling paradigms have continued to hamper meaningful dialogue between the two groups. Clinical ecologists are not found in allergy departments in medical schools. Their articles seldom appear in premier allergy journals—many times, but not always, because the articles fall short of recognized standards for scientific publications. Peer review in medicine may have both positive and negative consequences (Horrobin 1990). It serves to ensure quality control but it may also deter innovation. In the United States clinical ecologists are absent from academic medicine. In contrast, the Robens Institute, University of Surrey, England, has given ecologist William Rea a chair in environmental medicine. An environmental unit has recently been established at the Beijing Union Medical School in China. In Ontario, the Ministry of Health is funding a $600,000 study of food sensitivities at the University of Toronto as a result of the Ontario study on chemical hypersensitivity.

Feeling shut out of allergy, Randolph and several other allergists founded the Society for Clinical Ecology in 1965 and opened its doors to family physicians, otolaryngologists, and other physicians interested or involved in the area. In 1984 the society changed its name to the American Academy of Environmental Medicine, much to the chagrin of allergists, toxicologists, and other academicians in environmental medicine. Membership in the academy has grown by 225 members in the last 2 years and presently totals 570 (Howard 1989). An examination leading to certification in Environmental Medicine is offered, but the specialty has not been recognized by the American Board of Medical Specialties.

Allergists continue to point to the scientific basis of their practice and their detailed knowledge of immune mechanisms. Clinical ecologists stress the importance of their clinical observations. To some degree, their conflicts are an extension of the traditional tension between academicians and clinicians—a tension that has served neither side well.

Unfortunately, these conflicts may result in adverse economic consequences for patients who are already frustrated by their illness and their attempts to gain help. Allergists successfully persuaded Medicare not to reimburse for provocation-neutralization therapies (the predominant therapy used by ecologists, which is discussed further in Chapter 3) for treating food allergies, and allergists are often asked to provide independent assessments to insurance carriers who are contesting workers' compensation claims for disability associated with chemical exposure. One prominent allergist we interviewed was distressed at finding himself "on

TABLE 1-2. Contrast Between Paradigms of Traditional Medicine and Ecologically Oriented Medicine

Aspect	Traditional Medicine[a]	Clinical Ecology
Focus/approach	Body-centered; diagnosis contingent upon laboratory or clinical findings; symptoms alone generally insufficient for diagnosis	Environmentally oriented; diagnosis based upon temporal relationship between symptoms and chemical/food exposure; testing by avoidance and reexposure, sublingual or cutaneous provocation
Stage at which disease is diagnosed	End-organ damage generally must be present	Diagnosis may be made prior to end-organ damage, i.e., in a subclinical or pre-morbid state
View of patient	Focus on bodily parts and their malfunction. The patient is sick.	Focus on patient's chemical exposures and dietary habits. The patient's environment is sick.
Specialization	Anatomically demarcated[b]	No specialties per se. Concept of specialties considered limiting because environmental exposure may provoke symptoms in several systems simultaneously.
History taking	Review of all body systems by more thorough primary care takers; organ-oriented by specialists. Limited emphasis on dietary factors except in certain diseases, e.g., obesity, diabetes, hypercholesterolemia. Minimal attention to environmental exposures (except smoking) unless issue raised by patient	The more thorough practitioners review symptoms involving each system and search for environmental contributors to patient's illness. Emphasis is placed upon dietary and exposure histories.
Therapies	Drugs, surgery	Avoidance of environmental and food incitants; "neutralization" of symptoms by giving small dose of incitants; nutritional supplements; "detoxification"

[a] Within traditional medicine, allergists are among the practitioners most skilled in exploring environmental factors relating to a patient's illness. They also appreciate multiple organ involvement. Differences between allergy and clinical ecology are summarized in Table 1-3.

[b] Patients become "trained" to limit their complaints to the specialist's organ of interest; thus they may not complain of a headache to their gynecologist or of a rash to their psychiatrist.

TABLE 1-3. Contrast Between Traditional Allergy and Clinical Ecology

Aspect	Traditional Allergy[a]	Clinical Ecology[a]
Focus	Search for environmental triggers for symptoms/disease	Same as allergists
Practice priorities (in terms of frequency of diagnosis/relative importance in their patient population)	1. Biological inhalants, e.g., pollen, dust mite, molds, etc. 2. Food sensitivities 3. Chemical incitants	1. Chemical incitants 2. Food sensitivities 3. Biological inhalants
Diagnostic approaches:		
Biological Inhalants	Skin tests using extracts of pollens, molds, etc. Sometimes in vitro testing.	Skin testing also but using techniques/extract concentrations that differ from allergists
Foods	Skin tests using food extracts or in vitro tests, but usually limited to IgE-mediated diseases, such as eczema. Some practitioners do use elimination diets and food challenges for diagnosis. Double-blind, placebo-controlled challenges preferred.	Elimination diet with removal of suspect foods (or fasting) for 4–7 days followed by feeding challenges; sublingual or cutaneous provocation-neutralization heavily relied upon by majority
Chemicals	Interest in patient's chemical exposures includes occupational asthma, chemical "irritants" that exacerbate asthma and contact dermatitis. Also drug allergies or adverse reactions to drugs. "Chemical testing" limited to: 1. Skin testing for drugs (especially penicillin) 2. Patch testing for contact dermatitis 3. Inhalation challenges in specially constructed exposure chambers by a few practitioners (usually related to disability cases)	Low-level, often subtle chemical exposures (e.g., gas heat, formaldehyde, off-gassing from particleboard) responsible for many diverse symptoms/diseases. Patient avoids incitants. Some practitioners use sublingual or cutaneous doses of certain chemicals to provoke and neutralize symptoms. A few practitioners perform inhalation challenges.

(continued)

23

Aspect	Traditional Allergy[a]	Clinical Ecology[a]
Therapies used	Avoidance where practical. Antihistamines, topical and systemic steroids, cromolyn, and other drugs. Immunotherapy.	Chemical, food incitants avoided to regain tolerance. Drugs generally are avoided because of potential to sensitize. Some use of pancreatic enzymes, oral cromolyn, transfer factor, nystatin for *Candida* (yeast) sensitivity, etc. "Neutralization" used by most. Rotary/elimination diets often using organically grown food. Detoxification using saunas.
Definition of allergy	Adverse reaction involving antigen-antibody or sensitized lymphocytes	Adverse reaction to a substance
View of multiple chemical sensitivities	Varies greatly but majority of patients felt to have psychiatric disorders or erroneous belief systems	Consequence of exceeding patient's capacity to adapt to total environmental load

[a] Practice styles vary widely and even overlap within these groups; e.g., some allergists treat for *Candida* hypersensitivity, and some ecologists use traditional skin testing methods and immunotherapy for inhalant allergies.

the wrong side" from the patient's perspective as a result of taking referrals from insurance carriers.

While conflicts and antagonisms continue between allergists and clinical ecologists, the fields of toxicology and epidemiology are expanding their recognition that chemicals are harmful at lower and lower levels (Ashford 1987). Both classical toxicology and epidemiology have been invaluable in studies involving a single cause resulting in a single effect. With synergism (multiplicative effects of several toxins) or multiple effects, scientific investigations are more difficult to conduct and interpret. Indeed, the design of epidemiological studies for the discovery of chemical sensitivity requires great care. Because such a variety of inducing substances and, subsequently, triggering substances seems to be involved, several mechanisms could be operating simultaneously, and the "disease" may not be the same in all cases. Performing retrospective epidemiological studies on chemically sensitive persons without carefully defining the group to be investigated may result in a dilution of the prevalence of significant health effects. Then again, stratifying groups too narrowly may not yield statistically significant findings.

Other difficulties may interfere with using epidemiology to detect significant health effects of chemical exposures in certain situations. Spengler and associates (1983a) enumerate some potential problems in using epidemiologic studies to discover health effects of nitrogen dioxide (NO_2) exposure upon residents of homes with gas cooking.

1. Some homes with gas stoves have very low levels of NO_2, as low as those with electric stoves. Such variability could weaken the association between health effects and pollutant categories.

2. Only a subset of the exposed group (those having gas stoves) may be affected by gas stove combustion products.

3. High, short-term, or "peak" concentrations of NO_2 could be the primary cause of health effects, so that only a certain percentage of gas-cooking homes would be at risk.

4. Pollutants other than NO_2 might be more important causes of health effects. If so, variations in these pollutants among gas fuels and over time would tend to weaken any observed effect.

5. Statistical correction for factors that correlate with NO_2, such as socioeconomic status, may interfere with observing health effects. For example, low-income families are more likely to use gas stoves for supplementary heating.

The problems encountered in using epidemiology to identify health effects of NO_2 apply to multiple chemical sensitivity, although one further difficulty may be involved in the case of chemical sensitivity; the *same* exposure may produce different health effects in different individuals. These obstacles may be overcome as more is understood about this problem and the exposures involved.

At present, the allergists do not identify with the clinical ecologists, even though the ecologists are concerned with "altered reactivity." The toxicologists and epidemiologists do not seek to establish communication with the ecologists, even though the ecologists share their concern about exposure to toxic substances. If the model employed by clinical ecologists offers any insight into a cause-and-effect relationship between environmental incitants and illness, its application will be seriously hampered by the present state of affairs. Randolph has called for strengthening the relationship between toxicology and clinical ecology. We believe that some tenets of clinical ecology at its best will contribute to a *dynamic toxicology,* that is, observing the effects of chemical incitants in real time as those effects evolve.

Magnitude and Nature of the Problem

Chemical sensitivity presents a challenging puzzle for the scientist, physician, and public policy decision-maker. The pieces of the puzzle include (1) observations of possible offending or triggering substances and health effects, and (2) plausible mechanisms, diagnostic approaches, and therapies. Although a definitive and accurate picture is yet to come, at this time the pieces—viewed collectively—provide sufficient evidence to conclude that chemical sensitivity does exist as a serious health and environmental problem and that public and private sector action is warranted at both the state and federal levels (see also Massachusetts 1989, p. 1). Just how large a problem exists is not known at this time. The National Academy of Sciences has suggested, without providing documentation, that approximately 15 percent of the population may experience "increased allergic sensitivity" to chemicals (National Research Council 1987). Subsequent clarification by the chairman of the 1987 NAS workshop revealed that this figure is based on occupational studies of hypersensitivity to chemicals where the hypersensitivity was considered immunologic in origin (Lebowitz 1990). Based on the increasing outbreaks of sick building syndrome, increased reporting of symptoms in contaminated communities to state health departments, increased recognition of problems in the industrial workplace, and the increasing numbers of physicians treating chemically related sensitivities, the existing evidence does suggest that chemical sensitivity is on the rise and could become a large problem with significant economic consequences related to the disablement of productive members of society.

CHAPTER 2

Key Terms and Concepts

Terminology

A wide array of names has been applied to the syndromes suffered by patients with heightened reactivity to chemicals (Table 2-1). Each name has specific implications regarding the underlying cause, mechanism, or manifestations of the disease, and they overlap. A major hindrance in achieving scientific respectability has been the difficulty in agreeing upon a definition for this condition (or conditions). Cullen (1987b) has emphasized the importance of establishing a uniform case definition before meaningful epidemiologic studies can be undertaken, but cautions, "However constructed, the goal of descriptive studies must be refinement of the diagnostic criteria, in particular the very tentative boundaries with other diagnostic entities such as allergic, anxiety, panic and post-traumatic stress disorders, and physiologic sequelae of central nervous system (CNS) intoxication or injury, especially by organic solvents." He acknowledges possible overlap among these entities and offers the following case definition:

> Multiple chemical sensitivities (MCS) is an acquired disorder characterized by recurrent symptoms, referable to multiple organ systems, occurring in response to demonstrable exposure to many chemically unrelated compounds at doses far below those established in the general population to cause harmful effects. No single widely accepted test of physiologic function can be shown to correlate with symptoms. (Cullen 1987a)

27

TABLE 2-1. Attributes of Names for Heightened Reactivity

Cause	Mechanism	Effect
Environmentally induced illness	Immunologic illness	Multiple chemical sensitivities (MCS)
	Immunotoxicity	
Chemically induced (or acquired) hypersuscepti-bility	Immune dysfunction	Multiple chemical sensitivity syndrome
	Immune dysregulation	
	Conditioned odor response	Chemical hypersensitivity syndrome
Chemically acquired immune deficiency syndrome (chemical AIDS)	Fear/anxiety	Universal allergy
	Mass psychogenic illness	20th-century illness
	Various psychiatric disorders	Total allergy syndrome
		Environmental allergy or illness
		Cerebral allergy
The petro-chemical problem		Environmental maladaptation syndrome
		Food and chemical sensitivity

This case definition, intended for epidemiological use, is intentionally narrow. Cullen excludes persons who react to substances no one else is aware of on the basis that such individuals may be delusional and excludes persons who have bronchospasm, vasospasm, seizures, or "any other reversible lesion" that can be identified and specifically treated. Clinical ecologists, however, would argue that persons with bronchospasm, vasospasm, seizures, and other illnesses excluded by Cullen may well have the chemical sensitivity problem. Each issue of the clinical ecologists' journal, *Clinical Ecology,* contains the following definition:

> Ecologic illness is a chronic multi-system disorder, usually polysymptomatic, caused by adverse reactions to environmental incitants, modified by individual susceptibility and specific adaptation. The incitants are present in air, water, food, drugs and our habitat.

Although the patients the clinical ecologists and Cullen see are demographically divergent, the definitions of their illnesses are remarkably alike. Both *describe* the chemically sensitive patient in similar terms. (See Chapter 1 for a discussion of sensitive populations.) However, what is sorely needed is an objective test that can be applied in each individual case to determine, incontrovertibly, whether a particular person has multiple chemical sensitivities.

Given the multitude of environmental exposures (both chemical and food) that allegedly can result in a seemingly endless array of physical and mental syndromes and the frequent absence of findings on routine physical examination, the practitioner who sees these patients with their divergent and unfamiliar litany of complaints is at great disadvantage in trying to diagnose the condition.

To circumvent this problem, we propose the following *operational* definition of multiple chemical sensitivity, a definition that is based upon environmental testing:

> The patient with multiple chemical sensitivities can be discovered by removal from the suspected offending agents and by rechallenge, after an appropriate interval, under strictly controlled environmental conditions. Causality is inferred by the clearing of symptoms with removal from the offending environment and recurrence of symptoms with specific challenge.

Challenges conducted for research purposes should be performed in a double-blind, placebo-controlled manner. This definition embodies the approach to discovering environmental causation that was developed by Theron Randolph. Randolph originated the idea of an environmental unit employing what he terms "comprehensive environmental control" as both a diagnostic *and* therapeutic tool for dealing with these patients. Briefly, this technique involves placing the patient in a specially constructed environment devoid of materials that off-gas; avoiding the use of drugs, cosmetics, perfume, synthetic fabrics, pesticides, and similar substances; and having the patient fast for a period of days until symptoms resolve. This initial period of avoidance and fasting requires approximately 4 to 7 days on the average. During this time, the patient exhibits withdrawal symptoms such as headache, malaise, irritability, or depression. At the end of this time, the patient's symptoms, if environmentally related, should clear, provided that end-organ damage has not occurred. Clinical ecologists say this clearing does occur in the vast majority of patients. At the end of this avoidance phase, the patient generally has a markedly lower pulse rate and an increased sense of well-being, as well as a resolution of symptoms. Drinking waters from a variety of sources also are tested to find one most compatible with the patient. Next, individual foods are reintroduced, one per meal, over a two- to -three-week period. Following this, the patient is placed on a rotating diet of "safe" foods (i.e., foods that did not provoke symptoms for that particular patient). Finally, the patient is challenged with very low levels (levels routinely encountered in daily living) of common chemicals. Those exposures, both food and chemical, that induce symptoms are to be avoided. (Comprehensive environmental control is discussed in more detail later in this chapter.)

We feel strongly that this operational definition is essential to resolving, once and for all, the debate about whether an individual's symptoms are or are not environmentally induced. An environmental unit is necessary for scientific validation of the concept of chemical sensitivity. Because of the expense and time required by patients and physicians alike, we are not arguing that the unit be used for all patients. Such stringent measures are not necessary for most patients. For severe cases, however, no alternative is available at present, and only from firsthand observation of hospitalized patients can physicians have the opportunity to understand this illness better. In time, as more clinical data on these patients accumulate, physicians may be able to diagnose this disorder on the basis of the patient's history and a few key laboratory tests. For now, reliance must be placed on rigorous study in an environmental unit. Ultimately a *phenomenological* definition may emerge that allows physicians to diagnose, at least tentatively, chemical sensitivity based on a history of a specific sensitizing event (such as a pesticide exposure) followed by evidence of chemical and food sensitivities, multisystem effects, improvement after avoidance of exposure, and similar experiences of persons with like histories.

The environmental unit is the gold standard against which all other diagnostic approaches and screening techniques should be measured. An environmental unit is necessary in more severe cases, such as those who have failed outpatient attempts at management or for patients with seizures, suicidal tendencies, incapacitating migraine headaches, arrhythmias, or other problems requiring continuous vigilance. However, most individuals can remain outpatients while they are guided through an elimination diet, avoidance of possible chemical incitants, and rechallenge with suspected offenders. In a later section, we discuss provocation-neutralization and other office-based techniques that have been adopted by clinical ecologists in order to screen for and treat this illness. An enormous number of diagnostic and therapeutic modalities have been proposed, many of them lacking scientific verification. The gold standard—comprehensive environmental control with the use of an environmental unit—must be separated from the "fool's gold" of some of the more outlandish and untested diagnostic and therapeutic modalities. That is not to say that certain of those approaches are not now efficacious or may not "pan out" in the future, but many await and need critical scientific appraisal.

One aspect of clinical ecology that has repelled many traditional practitioners is the hodgepodge of unscientific, sometimes "new age," and even spiritual approaches patients with this illness have resorted to in a desperate struggle to restore their health. Randolph himself has expressed dismay at this turn of events. A survey of arthritis patients, who (like the chemically sensitive patient) have limited therapeutic options and may lead constricted life-styles, revealed that 94 percent had tried at least one unorthodox therapy (Wasner et al. 1980). From the chemically sensitive patient's viewpoint, searching for alternative therapies is understandable because the available treatments for this problem primarily have been avoidance of exposure and an elimination diet. Restrictive diets and avoidance do not permit full engagement in a modern life-style, and naturally patients seek alternatives. To the outside observer, these patients' practices appear cultist, and members of this supposed cult have been labeled in print as "true believers" and their physicians as "gurus" or "pseudoscientists." We find such terminology unfortunate and counterproductive. It would not appear to reflect the level of intelligence and professional achievements of these patients, many of whom are scientists, physicians, lawyers, teachers, and others from whom one would expect a modicum of common sense. Many are intelligent individuals who are angry at traditional medical practitioners for their unwillingness to study and understand this illness.

As individuals with chemical sensitivities are caught up in the escalating debate among medical practitioners, they find it more and more difficult to obtain unbiased, useful information regarding their condition. This difficulty underscores the importance of the operational definition we have proposed for chemical sensitivity. This definition takes the problem seriously and offers the environmental unit as the objective, scientific means for its study. With regard to other definitions that have been proposed, we agree that Cullen's narrow, descriptive case definition may have utility in some epidemiological investigations, for example, in tight-building syndrome or certain occupational outbreaks. In dealing with such a diversity of agents causing equally diverse effects at extraordinarily low levels with no true unexposed control group, however, such a definition may make engaging in meaningful epidemiologic investigations difficult.

Another term in this controversy that has confused patients and physicians alike is the word *allergy*. In a scholarly review, Alsoph Corwin (1985) of Johns Hopkins discusses the historical consequences that have arisen out of what he calls a faulty definition of *allergy*. He traces the evolution of the term and its consequences for the development of the field.

> Essentially, the fallacy lies in the confusion of hypersensitivity with immunity and the consequent exclusion from consideration of those cases of hypersensitivity which do not exhibit serological abnormalities.

These include many food reactions, drug allergies and reactions to environmental pollutants.

Corwin acknowledges Randolph and other clinical ecologists for not having been hamstrung by the limited definition of allergy as IgE-mediated (atopic) disease and for having attempted to document and elucidate the mechanisms of individual hypersensitivity, a problem he describes as much more prevalent than atopy. According to Corwin, "Estimates of the incidence of hypersensitivity in the general population run from 50-90%, whereas only approximately 6% have atopic allergy." The faulty definition of allergy, by excluding most hypersensitivities, has had devastating consequences, according to Corwin. He points to the work of Randolph in establishing cause-and-effect relationships between environmental factors and disease, saying, "Exclusion of these phenomena [that is, restricting the definition of allergy to IgE-mediated disease] also involves the world in tremendous expenditures for research for the elucidation of disease states when the solutions to the problems lie unused in the great medical libraries of the world." (See Chapter 3 and the Health Effects Appendix.) Here Corwin is alluding to the writings of Randolph and others.

The field of allergy and immunology today embraces antigen-antibody interactions (including those involving IgE), sensitized lymphocytes, and anaphylactoid drug reactions whose mechanisms remain obscure. Nevertheless, the view of allergy as primarily concerned with IgE-mediated phenomena has prevailed and has had considerable consequences for the practicing traditional allergist. William T. Kniker (the 1985 Bela Schick Lecturer, a professional honor bestowed by the American College of Allergy and Immunology) described the erosion of the allergist's practice by ear, nose, and throat (ENT) physicians, pulmonary specialists, and other groups. Kniker (1985) warned his fellow allergists: "We are not yet comfortable with other hypersensitivity diseases (immunologically triggered or not), adverse reactions to foods and environmental factors (occupational, hobby, home). . . . The narrowness of our specialty makes us extremely vulnerable." He quoted the author of *Megatrends*, who forecast "the triumph of the new paradigm of wellness, preventive medicine, and holistic care over the old model of illness, drugs, surgery, and treating symptoms, rather than the whole person. *The next big shift will be to focus on the environmental influences on health!*" (emphasis by Kniker).

Randolph (1987, p. 292) estimates that nearly 2,000 physicians, including roughly 900 ENT physicians, are applying the techniques of clinical ecology, in contrast to 3,000 to 3,500 conventional allergists.

Many communities have a surfeit of traditional allergists, and new allergists find demand for their skills waning (Kniker 1985). In contrast, clinical ecologists are quite busy. Randolph (1987) notes "when there were only a few of us we were treated as gadflies. Now that we are 40% of the total we are perceived as a real threat and dealt with accordingly." Almost all of the traditional allergists we interviewed feel strongly that allergy should embrace patients who have heightened reactivity to chemicals and/or foods, irrespective of the etiology of their problem. Selner (1985b), in particular, has written:

> There is every indication that the problem of chemical intolerance will continue to grow. We view these events as an opportunity for Allergy to appropriately expand its interest and influence into areas to which the public and the medical profession have traditionally turned to allergists for answers. . . . Although this may require fundamental changes in traditional practice priorities as well as allergy training curriculums, we believe the future of allergy practice can be found within this challenge.

Doris Rapp, a board-certified allergist who practiced traditional allergy for 18 years, turned to clinical ecology 14 years ago when she observed a dramatic reaction to food in a friend and became intrigued that clinical ecologists almost never placed asthmatic patients on steroids. She feels it is "ludicrous" to say that what ecologists do is not allergy. In her view (1985) she always was, still is, and will continue to be an allergist:

> I am doing the same things, for example, that I did for the first 18 years, but much better. I use the same extracts to test and treat. What I do, however, requires much more time, and the overhead is discouragingly increased. But the rewards are that patients, not helped by others, or previously not helped by myself, often get well quickly.

Ironically, patients with chemical sensitivity who have seen traditional allergists for what they felt was an "allergy" to tobacco smoke or some other substance have been lectured to on the subject of allergy and what its definition *really* is, that is, IgE-related disease. Some allergists we interviewed told us they attempt to educate these patients by handing them "Clinical Ecology" or "Controversial Techniques," the position papers of the American Academy of Allergy and Immunology (see references). Patients who consult allergists probably do not care whether what they have is, by definition, an allergy or not; what they are interested in is help in treating an adverse reaction to some substance.

Adaptation

One of the difficulties the observer encounters in trying to understand multiple chemical sensitivity is the ostensible lack of a central concept or unifying theory. Such a unifying theory does exist and revolves around the concept of adaptation, known in other contexts as *acclimation* or *acclimatization, habituation, developing tolerance* and even *addiction* (which we will explain later). Randolph has used the terms *adaptation* and *addiction* most often. However, reference to one of the other words may make grasping the concept easier. *Acclimatization* is a widely used term in occupational health that refers to workers gradually becoming accustomed to exposures on the job, for example, heat stress. Understanding adaptation is important here for two reasons: (1) adaptation makes difficult the discovery of the effects of a particular exposure on the body and (2) chemical exposures may adversely impact adaptation mechanisms and thus lead to illness.

Relatively little can be discovered about physiological "adaptation" by reading medical textbooks or recent major medical journals, in part because of the absence of Randolph's writings from such publications for a quarter of a century. However, detailed discussions of adaptation appear in all of Randolph's books, in journal articles by him from the 1950s, and in the clinical ecologists' literature. Our impression from interviewing traditional allergists is that many allergists are not aware of this concept and its potential clinical ramifications.

Concerning adaptation (or acclimation), Randolph (1962, p. 5) wrote:

> Human ecology embodies the concept of a person's adaptation to the conditions of his existence. The ecologic effects of chemical incitants are observed most advantageously by first isolating an individual from the *total chemical environment* and then observing his response to *re-exposure* to previously avoided *parts* of it.

That human beings respond to chronic exposure to environmental challenges by adapting, acclimating, acclimatizing, or even becoming addicted is widely recognized for a variety of substances. Most would agree that the use of narcotics, alcohol, nicotine, and even caffeine can be addicting. For example, the first cigarette ever smoked might be associated with eye and throat irritation, but over time, with more cigarettes, most individuals adapt, and primarily the pleasurable effect of nicotine on the brain are experienced. After months or years, more cigarettes (or alcohol or caffeine or drugs) may be required for the same amount of lift. The individuals may exhibit addictive behavior seeking cigarettes more frequently. Subsequently, quitting cigarettes (alcohol, caffeine, or drugs) may lead to withdrawal symptoms including irritability, drowsiness, fatigue, moodiness, and headache. After individuals have quit smoking, they may find themselves supersensitive to others' smoke (the forgotten eye and throat irritation reappear after a period of avoidance). This example parallels the food and chemical adaptation and addiction that ecologists like Randolph have described in their patients: frequent exposure to a substance results in adaptation (irritation and other warning signals may disappear); continued exposure may lead to addiction; reduction or cessation of exposure generally results in withdrawal symptoms.

The difference between chemical exposures and cigarettes, alcohol, or caffeine is that in the former case addiction is an unwitting process. The individual may have no idea it is occurring. But if the offending chemical is removed, withdrawal symptoms may ensue (Table 2-2). With reexposure to the substance following a period of avoidance, symptoms return, often quickly and much more obviously related to the exposure. What confuses many patients and practitioners is that the symptoms for which the individual is most likely to seek a physician's help are those that occur during withdrawal when the person is no longer exposed (or less exposed) to the offending agent! Thus headaches may occur when the individual smokes *fewer* cigarettes than usual or drinks *less* caffeine. Indeed, these unpleasant withdrawal symptoms may be forestalled by smoking another cigarette or taking another drink of coffee or alcohol and thus perpetuating addiction. Patients may report that smoking a cigarette or drinking a cup of coffee in the morning (after 8 or so hours without) *relieves* their headache (a withdrawal symptom) and they feel better, not suspecting that the cigarette or coffee might also be the cause of their headache.

Occupational health presents many examples in which acclimatization, inurement, or tolerance to a substance is known to develop, for example, exposure to ozone, nitroglycerin, cotton dust, welding fumes (containing zinc), and solvents. Note that the incitants mentioned thus far are all quite different from one another: some are ingestants, others inhalants; some are solid, others liquid or gaseous in form; some are organic, others inorganic; some (ozone) are simple inorganic molecular gases, whereas others (welding fumes) are complex mixtures of organic and inorganic substances in solid, liquid, and gaseous phases. The point is that the human organism has the capacity to adapt to an endless array of substances. In the extreme, as described for cigarettes and caffeine, individuals unknowingly may become *addicted* to the incitant, for exam-

TABLE 2-2. Stimulatory and Withdrawal Symptoms Associated with Exposure to Various Foods and Chemicals[a]

Behavior Classification	Response Classifications	Stimulatory Level	Response Characteristics	Typical Responses
Stimulated	Maladapted Cerebral and Behavioral Responses	+ + + +	MANIC, WITH OR WITHOUT CONVULSIONS	Distraught, excited, agitated, enraged, and panicky. Circuitous or one-track thoughts, muscle-twitching and jerking of extremities, convulsive seizures, and altered consciousness may develop.
		+ + +	HYPOMANIC, TOXIC, ANXIOUS AND EGOCENTRIC	Aggressive, loquacious, clumsy (ataxic), anxious, fearful, and apprehensive; alternating chills and flushing, ravenous hunger, excessive thirst. Giggling or pathological laughter may occur.
	Adapted Responses	+ +	HYPERACTIVE, IRRITABLE, HUNGRY, AND THIRSTY	Tense, jittery, "hopped-up," talkative, argumentive, sensitive, overly responsive, self-centered, hungry, and thirsty; flushing, sweating, and chilling may occur, as well as insomnia, alcoholism, and obesity.
		+	STIMULATED BUT RELATIVELY SYMPTOM-FREE	Active, alert, lively, responsive, and enthusiastic, with unimpaired ambition, energy, initiative, and wit. Considerate of the views and actions of others. This usually comes to be regarded as "normal" behavior.
"Normal"		0	BEHAVIOR ON AN EVEN KEEL, AS IN HOMEOSTASIS	Calm, balanced, level-headed reactions. Children expect this from their parents and teachers. Parents expect this from their children. We all expect this from our associates.

Withdrawal (maladapted) responses: loss of tolerance

Maladapted Localized Responses	−	LOCALIZED ALLERGIC MANIFESTATIONS	Running or stuffy nose, clearing throat, coughing, wheezing. Asthma, itching (eczema and hives), gas, diarrhea, constipation (colitis), urgency and frequency of urination, and various eye and ear syndromes.
Maladapted Systemic Responses	− −	SYSTEMIC ALLERGIC MANIFESTATIONS	Tired, dopey, somnolent, mildly depressed, edematous with painful syndromes (headache, neckache, backache, neuralgia, myalgia, myositis, arthralgia, arthritis, arteritis, chest pain), and cardiovascular effects.[b]
Maladapted Advanced Stimulatory Responses	− − −	BRAIN-FAG, MILD DEPRESSION, AND DISTURBED THINKING	Confused, indecisive, moody, sad, sullen, withdrawn, or apathetic. Emotional instability and impaired attention, concentration, comprehension, and thought processes (aphasia, mental lapse, and blackouts).
	− − − −	SEVERE DEPRESSION, WITH OR WITHOUT ALTERED CONSCIOUSNESS	Unresponsive, lethargic, stuporous, disoriented, melancholic, incontinent, regressive thinking, paranoid orientation, delusions, hallucinations, sometimes amnesia and coma.

[a] Begin at 0 (normal behavior, feeling well), and follow the stimulated levels (+ up to + +, + + +, etc.) which result from exposure to a particular substance (tolerance or adaptation is occurring during these stages). With removal from exposure, the individual withdraws (+ + +, down to + +, +, 0, −, + −, − −, etc.) and experiences symptoms of withdrawal (loss of tolerance, or maladaptation).

[b] Cardiovascular manifestations, including rapid or irregular pulse, hypertension, phlebitis, anemia, and bleeding and bruising tendencies, may occur at any level.

Source: Randolph, T. and Moss, R., *An Alternative Approach to Allergies,* copyright J. B. Lippincott Co., Philadelphia, PA (1980).

ple, to some solvents. Addiction is most likely to be recognized for substances that have euphoric or other pleasant properties and less likely to be recognized for chemicals and foods without these properties.

By isolating his patients from their usual environments and then reexposing them to various foods and chemicals one by one, Randolph discerned that adaptation plays an important role in many common substances people eat, drink, or inhale. Virtually any food or chemical follows the same pattern: initially, the individual notes symptoms when the substance is first encountered; gradually, with continued exposure or multiple reexposures, tolerance or adaptation or acclimatization occurs. "Addiction" to commonly eaten foods, such as corn, wheat, milk, eggs, and citrus fruit, and to common chemical inhalants, for example, formaldehyde or gas combustion products, although generally not recognized by patients or their physicians, also occurs, according to ecologists.

As we indicated earlier, what Randolph contributed was a systematic approach to studying individual responses to foods and chemicals. By removing individuals from their total background of environmental incitants and exposing them to each food and each chemical individually, he was able to observe a biphasic response to some of these substances (Fig. 2-1). He noted that initially the individual might experience a stimulatory effect (adapted response; tolerance develops) lasting varying periods of time depending upon the incitant. However, this "up" phase was generally followed by a withdrawal phase (maladapted response; loss of tolerance). Upon beginning to experience unpleasant withdrawal symptoms, the individual would seek, consciously or unconsciously, more of the same substance. These ups and downs follow a sort of sinusoidal (biphasic) pattern, as depicted in Figure 2-1. On the graph, beginning at zero, the patient is free of symptoms and at baseline health status. Following a one-time or occasional exposure to a provoking substance, stimulatory effects result; after a period of time (minutes to hours to days, depending upon the nature of the incitant), the stimulatory effects subside and give way to withdrawal symptoms. The frequency of these up and down reactions depends upon the frequency of the person's contact with the incitant. The amplitude of the stimulatory and withdrawal portions of the reaction depends upon the substance and the individual's susceptibility (degree of adaptation or addiction) to it. The particularly sensitive person exhibits larger amplitudes than the normals. For example, an occasional drinker or a painter exposed to solvents the first few times might have a relatively pleasant up phase with relatively few withdrawal symptoms afterward. As exposures become more frequent, however, addiction may occur. A painter might visit other painters on his day off in order to "sniff" some solvent. (Ran-

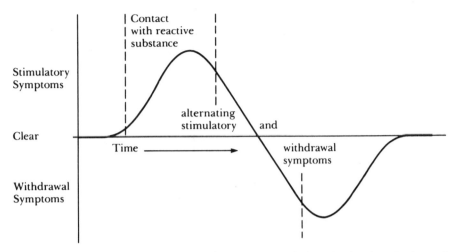

FIGURE 2-1. *Symptom progression of a single reaction to an incitant. During the early phases of exposure to a particular substance, stimulatory symptoms predominate ("up," "hyper," jittery). As exposure to the offending agent continues, adaptation occurs and fewer of these symptoms are experienced. With removal from (or discontinuance of) exposure, the individual experiences withdrawal symptoms ranging in intensity from mild to severe. (From O'Banion, D. R.,* Ecological and Nutritional Treatment of Health Disorders, *1981, p. 68. Courtesy of Charles C Thomas, Publisher, Springfield, Illinois.)*

dolph 1987, p. 109); perhaps drinking alcohol has a role in forestalling solvent withdrawal symptoms in some susceptible painters.

The key to understanding multiple chemical sensitivity may lie in recognizing these ups and downs that occur after exposure to many different substances. Table 2-2 illustrates the pattern of reaction Randolph claims he has observed in thousands of patients after exposure to an incitant. The amplitude of a reaction varies from person to person and incitant to incitant, but the pattern is quite constant. Beginning in the center of the table at zero, read upward for stimulatory effects and downward for withdrawal effects. Note that many of the stages, both stimulatory and withdrawal, are characterized by central nervous system (CNS) symptoms such as anxiety, confusion, depression, and irritability. Such symptoms are commonly noted by patients with multiple chemical sensitivities. The early stimulated (+ and + +) levels are adaptive responses by the body to an environmental incitant. Individuals at adaptation level + are stimulated but relatively free of symptoms. They may remain at this relatively desirable level (which often is confused with normalcy, level 0) indefinitely. According to Randolph, individuals rarely seek medical help at levels +, or + +. However, the onset of withdrawal (−) symptoms, whether systemic (fatigue, myalgia, or impaired concentration) or localized (rhinitis, asthma, or colitis), brings patients to the doctor. Often, the plus phase of any reaction is followed by a minus phase at least as intense, or perhaps one stage deeper. Thus a + + stimulatory phase may be followed by a − − or − − − withdrawal phase (see Table 2-2). In many individuals, every step of the entire sinusoidal progression of symptoms (for example, +, + +, +, 0, −, − −, − − − and finally back up to − −, −, and 0) can be observed. The most extreme case would be progression from mania to deep depression in a single patient, as in manic-depressive disease. Another interesting aspect is the tendency for psychotic (+ + + + or − − − −) and classical allergic (− and − −) manifestations to alternate in individuals. In the 1800s Savage described several cases in which insanity alternated with asthma; when one was present, the other disappeared. Old psychiatric texts refer to this vacillation between physical and mental manifestations as *alternation* (Randolph 1976b).

With long-term exposure to a given incitant (for instance, alcohol), especially in certain individuals, the degree and duration of stimulation may become less and less while the withdrawal or depressed phase becomes deeper and more prolonged. At face value, this sinusoidal reaction to a substance might seem a somewhat artificial construct, but Randolph asserts it is not. Randolph himself has hospitalized, fasted, and tested more than 10,000 people with many foods and chemicals since 1956, and his theories are distilled from observations of patients who have gone through an environmental unit (Randolph 1980, p. 169). For a patient with sensitivities involving foods alone, an elimination diet or fasting followed by reintroduction of single foods may be adequate for diagnosis. However, Randolph states that since World War II he has observed increasing numbers of individuals who respond adversely to the chemical environment. Subtle chemical sensitivities may be difficult to assess while a patient remains at home or even in most hospitals because these places generally contain background low levels of natural gas, disinfectants, perfumes, cleaners, tobacco smoke, paints, varnishes, adhesives, and other substances. According to Randolph, the patient's symptoms may be *masked* by the presence of these contaminants (more on this subject follows later).

With regard to chemical sensitivity (or *susceptibility*, a term Randolph prefers in order to avoid confusion with classical, IgE-mediated allergic sensitivity), Randolph (1987, p. 78) notes that, more than foods, chemical exposures are:

> associated with higher degrees of individual susceptibility and relatively greater persistence of susceptibility as well as more advanced clinical syndromes. Also, once individual susceptibility to one or a few environ-

mental chemical exposures has developed, it almost invariably tends to spread to involve other combustion products and derivatives of gas, oil and coal.

Randolph has referred to this as the "petrochemical problem." The stimulatory and withdrawal levels for foods and chemicals overlap each other (Fig. 2-2) so that in real life—outside an environmental unit—at any given moment what the organism is feeling is a summation of all effects, whether stimulatory or depressive, of all substances inhaled, contacted, or ingested. Figure 2-2 shows that attempts to identify the effects of single substances would be frustrated by the overlapping responses. Only by placing the individual in an environment devoid of chemical and food incitants is one able to determine whether the illness is alleviated. Assuming the patient improves (which occurs in the majority of cases, according to ecologists), the next step is to reexpose the person to individual substances in order to avoid overlapping responses and then to observe the result. According to Randolph, only in this way can the stimulatory and withdrawal phases associated with a given substance be discerned. If all possible food and chemical contributors are not removed, an effect may be missed. Hence, in order to rule out environmental illness definitively, an environmental unit would be required. An environmental illness could be ruled in on an outpatient basis, but not ruled out. However, environmental factors should be ruled out before psychiatric diagnoses and labels are applied to patients (see later discussion on psychogenic mechanisms).

In real life, following several days' avoidance of suspected incitants, a very robust response may occur with re-exposure, but not be recognized as such: An asthmatic might feel well after spending a week in a Caribbean island, breathing clean air and eating a diet devoid of usual foods, only to have a severe, life-threatening asthmatic response to exhaust from the engine of a boat taking the individual home. Once

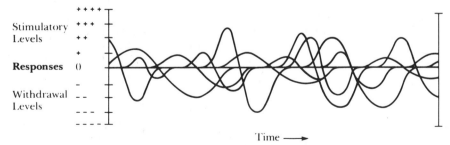

FIGURE 2-2. Overlapping of responses to food and chemical incitants in an individual with multiple exposures and multiple chemical sensitivities.

the asthmatic readapts, acclimatizes to auto exhaust combustion products and other air pollutants in the area, and experiences only chronic wheezing. Thus, following deadaptation (removal of incitants), the individual exhibits a more acute and convincing reaction upon reexposure. This appears to be what occurs in an environmental unit during testing. So acute and convincing are some of these reactions that patients themselves erroneously (at least in the eyes of some) surmise they must have an "allergy" to a particular substance. However, if the patient is not deadapted (unmasked) when tested, a reaction may not occur, convincing the physician that the "allergy" was all in the patient's mind. Many double-blind studies by allergists and others in the past have not taken this phenomenon of masking into account and therefore may be flawed. The sensitivity, if not tested for in the unmasked state, may easily be missed.

Occupational health has many widely recognized examples of adaptation that are analogous. They, too, fit a biphasic pattern. Industrial hygienists and occupational health physicians know that one of the most valuable clues to work-related illness is a history of intense symptoms following return to work *after* a vacation or weekend (leading to withdrawal and deadaptation). The following examples help underscore the existence of this phenomenon of adaptation. These particular examples may or may not also represent multiple chemical sensitivity. Individuals who are more sensitive or susceptible to the following substances may be the same individuals who are prone to developing multiple chemical sensitivities. In other words, multiple chemical sensitivities may reflect failure of adaptation in some sense. Failure may be the result of individual tendencies, an environmental insult, or some combination of the two. Bearing in mind that multiple chemical sensitivity might be what is actually occurring in the most sensitive subgroups exposed to these substances, let us now turn to some specific examples from occupational medicine:

1. Welding on galvanized metal causes evolution of zinc oxide fumes that, when inhaled, provoke an influenza-like syndrome with headaches, nausea, weakness, myalgia, coughing, dyspnea, and fever. The same symptoms may result from inhaling fumes of copper, magnesium, aluminum, and other metals. Hunter (1978, p. 407) writes:

   > The frequency and severity of the attacks are affected by the regularity of exposure for those who work continuously in the trade seem to acquire a tolerance which, however, is only transient, since it may be lost during a weekend away from work. In such cases the relapse of symptoms after working on a Monday gives rise to the name "Monday Fever."

Removal from exposure (deadaptation) for a couple of days is followed by an exacerbation of symptoms upon return to work.

2. Cotton (Hunter 1978, pp. 1043–1045), grain, and other organic dusts, as well as vapors from contaminated humidifiers, also produce an acute flulike illness, usually on the first workday after a period away from the job. In other words, after a period of deadaptation, reexposure to organic dust or vapors may provoke acute symptoms. In this example and the previous one, systemic symptom (metal fume fever and flulike illness from organic dust exposure), appear, not just respiratory symptoms. Flulike symptoms involving multiple systems occur in a subgroup of exposed workers. Although the physiological responses to metal fumes and organic dusts have been characterized and differ markedly from that of other substances discussed here, nevertheless there is an adaptive component to these responses. Adaptation appears to be an attribute of many, if not all, physiological systems.

3. Nitroglycerin, used to manufacture gunpowder, rocket fuels, and dynamite, may cause severe headaches, breathing difficulty, weakness, drowsiness, nausea, and vomiting as a result of inhalation. Lesser symptoms may appear with oral administration (for example, as a drug for cardiac patients) or skin contact. Even wives of nitroglycerin workers who launder and iron their husbands' clothing may experience similar symptoms, headache being the most prominent.

> The headache may continue for one or two hours, or even for three or four days. The onset may be associated with exhilaration, but usually this passes and the victim becomes depressed. . . . Tolerance to exposure develops after three or four days of continued exposure, but is lost after two days away from work. Since the 19th century, workers have been known to avoid the Monday headache, once they become tolerant to nitroglycerin, by placing nitroglycerin under their hatbands over the weekend, or sucking occasionally on a piece of dynamite. Others inhaled the fumes from their work clothes over the weekend (Daum 1983, pp. 639, 648).

Stimulatory (exhilaration) and withdrawal (depression) symptoms occur in a biphasic manner. Alcohol may make dynamite headaches worse and cause confusion, extreme agitation, hallucinations, or violent behavior; individuals have even been known to commit murder (Daum 1983). Here then is an example of an individual exposed to a particular chemical who exhibits reduced tolerance for an ingestant.

Most studies have failed to show a difference in blood pressure between dynamite workers and controls; however, differences are noted between measurements taken in dynamite workers on Monday (lower) and those taken later in the week. Without insight into the principles of adaptation, one might overlook or discount such a phenomenon and examine only the average blood pressure during the week. Nitroglycerin has other effects on the central nervous system such as mania (+ + + +), epilepsy (+ + + +), depression (− −, − − −, − − − −), aphasia (− − −), parasthesias (− −), and headaches (− −). Understanding adaptation, one could trace all of these symptoms through their stimulatory and withdrawal levels.

Noteworthy is a study by the Pennsylvania Department of Health of dynamite workers who suffered sudden death that was felt to be cardiovascular in origin (Carmichael et al. 1963). Almost all of them died after a period away from exposure on the job, that is, during the withdrawal phase (see footnote to Table 2-2 regarding cardiovascular manifestations). Most of these workers were 30 to 45 years old, and their physical exams were largely unremarkable. "Monday morning angina" has been described among dynamite workers; if their angina attack does not interfere, returning to work may cure it! The incidence of sudden death among workers at one dynamite plant was 15 times the expected rate. The mechanism is unknown; however, some have speculated that acclimatization followed by vasospasm on withdrawal from exposure suggests an increased sympathetic nervous system output compensatory mechanism (Daum 1983). William Rea, a cardiothoracic surgeon and ecologist, has written extensively concerning arrhythmias and coronary vasospasm—both of which he feels may contribute to sudden death—resulting from food and/or chemical sensitivities (Rea 1981, 1987b).

Hunter relates the story of a dynamite worker who had severe headaches and whose wife and children had terrible headaches as well. His physician recommended slipping two or three grains of powder under his hatband and taking a few more grains and hiding them around the house. This advice worked well; their headaches disappeared. However, anyone who came to the house as a visitor would get "a hell of a headache." Alfred Nobel, inventor of dynamite and founder of the Nobel prize, likewise suffered from dynamite headaches over many years. Hunter notes that individual susceptibility to nitroglycerin varies tremendously. In all but 2 to 3 percent of workers, tolerance is acquired within a few days of exposure (Hunter 1978, pp. 560–566). Conceivably, those who fail to develop tolerance to nitroglycerin may have the chemical susceptibility (multiple chemical sensitivity) problem.

4. Ozone, an air pollutant of special concern to residents of Los Angeles and other cities, has been the focus of considerable research relevant to adaptation. Intrigued by how little respiratory illness and death

occurred relative to the high levels of ozone in very polluted cities and suspecting adaptation might play a protective role, Hackney and associates (1977a) compared the responses of four Canadians (not adapted) and four Californians (adapted) to ozone challenges. Although reactivity varied greatly from individual to individual, Californians were only minimally reactive to levels that for the Canadians caused coughing, substernal discomfort and airway irritation, pulmonary function test decrements, and increased red blood cell fragility.

In another experiment, six volunteers with respiratory hyperreactivity were placed in an environmental chamber with ozone at 0.5 ppm (parts per million), typical of ambient levels, for 4 days (Hackney et al. 1977b). Five of six had decreased pulmonary function during days 1 to 3, but gradually improved, almost to baseline by day 4, suggesting adaptation had occurred. The authors note that not all adverse effects of ozone may be prevented by adaptation; for example, increased blood cell fragility may persist. Therefore, adaptation or masking of some symptoms may occur while other physiological alterations continue.

Individuals' abilities to adapt to ozone appear to depend upon their initial sensitivity to it. More sensitive persons adapt more slowly and cannot maintain the adaptation as long; they usually remain adapted less than 7 days following cessation of exposure (Horvath 1981).

Adaptation to ozone seems to be a concentration-dependent phenomenon. Chronic exposure to low levels of ozone in the air does not mitigate the effects of acute exposures to ozone at higher concentrations (Gliner 1983). These observations pertaining to ozone might also apply to the exposure experiences of chemically sensitive patients.

Because some tolerance to ozone can be induced in small rodents exposed to 1 ppm of ozone in as little as one hour, Stokinger (1965) speculated that the mechanism that seemed to explain observations in animals best was "either a cellular depletion phenomenon or enzyme stimulation." Mustafa and Tierney (1978), discussing oxygen (as opposed to ozone) toxicity caution, "the term 'tolerance' should not be considered to indicate absolute tolerance, because continuing injury does occur, and eventually, emphysema-like changes and fibrosis develop"; in the short term, tolerance may be protective, but "when exposures are continuous or intermittent for a period of weeks or even years, it is likely that unacceptable lung injury is necessary to keep the mechanism of tolerance or adaptation activated." With regard to ozone exposures among "adapted" Southern Californians, Mustafa and Tierney comment, "Whether or not they have continuing lung injury with increased probability of bronchitis, emphysema, or even malignancy is not known, although some reports have supported the concept."

Bell and King (1982), extending these ideas to chemically sensitive patients, speculate that their chronic symptoms "may reflect the more insidious, non-adapting changes induced by offending foods and chemicals. At the same time, the more obvious and dramatic adverse clinical effects may be masked or adapted."

5. Solvents are among the chemicals most frequently implicated by chemically sensitive patients who attribute the onset of their illness to a particular exposure (Terr 1989a; Cone et al. 1987; see Table 2-3). Vapors from various solvents are the most prevalent of indoor air contaminants (Molhave 1982). The volatile organic compounds (VOCs) associated with sick building syndrome are in large part solvent vapors. The sensory irritation, headache, drowsiness, and other symptoms noted by occupants of tight buildings are consistent with known effects of solvent vapors, albeit at much higher concentrations. *Solvent* is a very broad term encompassing a wide range of liquids that are capable of dissolving or dispersing other substances. They are found in many products commonly used at home and at work, for example, in paint, varnishes, adhesives, pesticides, and cleaning solutions.

The adverse short- and long-term effects of solvents are widely recognized by occupational health professionals. In recent years much effort has been directed toward reducing the solvent content of paints by using larger fractions of water as a vehicle for pigments and thereby reducing exposures for persons applying them. Nevertheless, exposures to solvents at home and at work may be significant, particularly in confined spaces or tightly sealed structures with inadequate fresh (outdoor) air for ventilation. Where solvents are applied over large surface areas, the opportunity for evaporation is increased, and the concentration of solvents in the air may reach high levels.

Those who have painted or used solvents to any major extent are well aware of the olfactory fatigue (nasal adaptation) that occurs and may have experienced the stimulatory and depressive properties of solvents. Alcoholic beverages contain the solvent ethanol, which has related and familiar stimulatory and withdrawal effects. A study of Finnish car painters demonstrated increased complaints of fatigue and nausea and reduced vigilance and concentration while at work (Husman 1980). Many (more than controls) reported they often felt excess tiredness after the workday (withdrawal). Inquiries to painters

TABLE 2-3. Causative Agent in Claims of Work-related Environmental Illness

Agent	Number	Agent	Number	Agent	Number
Paint, thinner	10	Carbon tetrachloride	2	Tar	1
Smoke	7	Paper	2	Wood dust	1
Organic solvents	7	Hair sprays	2	Beet sugar dust	1
Pesticides	6	Office machines	2	Detergent	1
Xylene	5	Photographic chemical	2	Nail polish	1
Phenol	5	New building	2	Polyurethane	1
Dust	5	Hydrogen	1	Soap	1
Formaldehyde	4	Helium	1	Germicide	1
"Chemicals"	4	Argon	1	Vehicle exhaust	1
New carpets	4	Nickel	1	Unspecified fumes	1
Ammonium compounds	4	Lead	1	Chairs	1
Freon	3	Ethanol	1	Heat at work	2
Solder flux	3	Nitric acid	1	Fall at work	2
Welding fumes	3	Sulfur dioxide	1	Stress at work	1
Fiberglas	3	Hydrochloric acid	1	Dry air	1
Perfumes	3	Polyvinyl chloride	1	Herpes zoster	1
Food	2	Toluene diisocyanate	1	Scabies	1
Hydrocarbons	2	Methylene chloride	1	Uncertain	2
Trichlorethane	2	Kerosene	1	None	5
Fuel	2	Glue	1		

Source: Terr, A., "Clinical Ecology in the Workplace," *Journal of Occupational Medicine* 31(3): 257–261, p. 258 (1989) (copyright American College of Occupational Medicine).

who had changed employment revealed that 52 of 101 had changed vocations and 26 of the 52, or half of those who had left car painting, mentioned health or other occupational hazards as reasons for leaving. This latter group reported having experienced a relatively high symptom frequency level while working at car painting. Thus workers who were sensitive to chemicals were more likely to migrate to other occupations, which could help to explain why chemically sensitive individuals are often seen among office workers or light industrial workers rather than among workers in heavy industry. Terr (1989a) summarized the occupations of 90 individuals referred to him for workers' compensation evaluation (Table 2-4). Migration of sensitive subgroups to other jobs or out of the workforce may contribute to the so-called healthy worker effect.

TABLE 2-4. Occupations of 90 Patients Claiming Work-related Environmental Illness

Occupation	Number	Occupation	Number
Office work		Education	
Clerical worker	12	Teacher	8
Telephone operator	4	Food industry	
Manager	2	Waitress	2
Salesperson	1	Baker	1
Transportation		Equipment mechanic	1
Flight attendant	6	Other manufacturing	
Mechanic	3	Lithographer	4
Pilot	2	Welder	1
Bus driver	1	Plastics worker	1
Train operator	1	Wood worker	1
Medicine and social work		Lumber worker	1
Nurse	4	Hairdresser	3
Social worker	2	Writer	2
X-ray technician	1	Engineer	2
Respiratory therapist	1	Dry cleaner	1
Psychotherapist	1	Carpet layer	1
Dental assistant	1	Security guard	1
Laboratory technician	1	Artist	1
Electronic manufacturing		Geologist	1
Assembler or technician	7	City dump operator	1
Solderer	3	Transformer repair	1
Tool and die maker	1	Fabric salesman	1
Research worker	1		

Source: Terr, A., "Clinical Ecology in the Workplace," *Journal of Occupational Medicine* 31(3): 257–261, p. 258 (1989) (copyright American College of Occupational Medicine).

Molhave (1982) identified chemicals emanating from 42 modern building materials, the ten most common of which were solvents (Table 2-5). Health effects most commonly involve the central nervous system. Molhave and associates (1986) exposed individuals who had previously complained of sick building syndrome symptoms to a mixture of 22 volatile organic compounds common in indoor air, predominantly solvents, for 2¾ hours. Levels were much lower than occupational health standards required and in the range of levels found in tight buildings. These healthy but sensitive subjects complained of nasal and throat irritation and inability to concentrate at levels of solvents far below permissible occupational exposure levels. (For a fuller discussion of Molhave's studies, see Chapter 3.) A similar study, using healthy subjects who had not previously complained of symptoms, showed no effect on the ability to concentrate (Otto et al. 1990).

Chemically sensitive patients commonly report central nervous system symptoms at solvent levels as low as those used by Molhave and lower. Their complaints are consistent with the recognized health effects of these substances, albeit the *levels* of exposure that trigger symptoms in these patients may be lower by orders of magnitude.

According to Randolph (1980), the stimulatory effects of solvents may be pleasant or unpleasant, depending upon the person and the exposure. At the + level (see Table 2-2), a normal individual exposed to solvents may experience being alert, enthusiastic, energetic, and witty

TABLE 2-5. Commonly Identified Chemicals Off-gassing from 42 Modern Building Materials

The 10 Most Frequently Identified Compounds	*The 10 Compounds in Highest Average Equilibrium Concentration*
Toluene	Toluene
n-Decane	3-Xylene
1,2,4-Trimethylbenzene	$C_{10}H_{16}$ (Terpene)
n-Undecane	n-Butyl acetate
3-Xylene	n-Butanol
2-Xylene	n-Hexane
n-Propyl benzene	4-Xylene
Ethyl benzene	Ethoxy ethyl acetate
n-Nonane	n-Heptane
1,3,5-Trimethyl benzene	2-Xylene

Source: Reprinted with permission from "Indoor Air Pollution Due to Organic Gases and Vapours of Solvents in Building Materials," in *Environmental International* 8:117–127, 122. Molhave, L., Moghisssi, A., and Moghissi, B. (eds.). Copyright 1982, Pergamon Press plc., Elmsford, NY.

and may sustain this level for long periods while a chemically sensitive person may progress quickly to + + and feel tense, jittery, argumentative, sensitive, and overly responsive and experience chills or flushing. Very sensitive individuals may become manic or develop seizures (+ + + +).

During withdrawal, symptoms for relatively healthy individuals may be only mild, localized symptoms (−) *resembling* an allergy, for example, a runny or stuffy nose, coughing, wheezing, eczema, hives, diarrhea, and eye and ear symptoms. However, the response is not actually an allergic one; there is no evidence that IgE plays a role. If withdrawal is more severe (− −), fatigue, depression, muscle and joint aches, headache, and a rapid or irregular heart rate may ensue. At more advanced stages in very sensitive individuals (− − −, − − − −), confusion, indecision, and apathy can occur with comprehension and concentration becoming impaired. The most severe stage (− − − −) may be attended by stupor, delusions, and hallucinations. From a clinical viewpoint, Randolph's model could serve as a useful framework for following the progression of these patients' symptoms. Many patients with chemical sensitivity seem to experience the more advanced stages of stimulation and depression in the model. According to Randolph, when they are deadapted and then exposed to a *single* incitant, the stepwise, sinusoidal progression up through stimulatory levels and back down through withdrawal levels can best be observed. In normal daily life, exposures overlap and discrete stages may not be discerned.

Studies of xylene, one of the most prevalent solvents in indoor air (see Table 2-5), conducted by Riihimaki and Savolainen (1980) demonstrate that its effects are attenuated as exposure continues, presumably due to adaptation. Their work is discussed in detail in Chapter 5.

We have mentioned a number of the exposures that are recognized as involving adaptation or addiction. No doubt the physiological events that allow us to adapt to the ozone are quite different from those for nicotine or nitroglycerine. Nevertheless, it is clear that human beings adapt to a wide variety of substances in their environment. What is not clear is the specific role adaptation plays in the dramatic responses patients with food and chemical sensitivities have to low-level exposures that do not overtly affect others (for further discussion of possible mechanisms, see Chapter 4).

Without exception, all traditional allergists we interviewed recognized the phenomenon of acclimatization or adaptation and agreed that it was potentially a crucial variable that should be controlled in studies of low-level exposure to chemicals. These concepts are familiar to occupational health practitioners and industrial hygienists because they observe such effects firsthand among workers exposed to chemicals. Randolph (1962, p. 7) states that most physicians see patients long after adaptation has occurred and at the time when end organ damage is setting in: "It is much as if the physician arrived at the theatre sometime during the last scene of the second act of a three act play—puzzled by what may have happened previously to the principal actor, his patient." Through comprehensive environmental control (that is, an environmental unit), one can overcome the masking effect of adaptation and back up or reverse the exposure to allow monitoring of toxicity in progress. The environmental unit represents a kind of *dynamic toxicology;* traditional medical approaches provide only a snapshot of what is happening to the patient.

The sheer heterogeneity of substances that can evoke adverse reactions (those enumerated above and others) suggests a fundamental mechanism of adaptation to environmental substances. The mechanism may involve the nervous system or some other system(s) rather than the immune system. However, the intense symptoms that may occur with deadaptation and reexposure resemble a classic allergic response, that is, an untoward reaction to an incitant. This concept has clinical utility.

Because adaptation appears to be a generalized response (Selye 1946), a toxic insult to, for example, the sympathetic nervous system or enzyme detoxification pathways could cause a general loss of the ability to adapt to a wide variety of substances, including other chemicals and even foods (the spreading phenomenon). Knowing the mechanism by which this occurs would, of course, be ideal. Thus far, it has eluded clinical ecologists and placed them at a distinct disadvantage.

Observing a phenomenon and documenting its existence must, of necessity, precede knowledge of its mechanism. Of course, knowing the mechanism of a disease is not necessary in order to prevent it. A historic example occurred in 1854 when a London physician, John Snow, noted that individuals who developed cholera obtained their drinking water from the Broad Street pump. Medical folklore tells us that by ordering the removal of the pump handle, he stopped the epidemic (Snow 1936). Not until 1883, almost 30 years later, did Koch discover the bacterium responsible for cholera. Analogous to the current dilemma, understanding the mechanism for food and chemical sensitivities is not necessary in order to begin diagnosing and treating them. Eventually, knowledge of the mechanism may suggest better treatments.

With regard to patients with chemical sensitivities who also develop dietary intolerances, Bell (1982, pp. 35–36) notes that "foods are not only sources of nutrients, but also complex mixtures of organic chemicals. For instance, it is the unique pattern of chemical constituents that make a tomato a tomato rather than an apple." She provides a partial listing of chemical constituents of tomato, apple, milk, and orange (see

Table 4-2). Allergists Butcher, Salvaggio and associates (1982) reported an interesting case of a worker with toluene di-isocyanate (TDI) sensitivity who was also intolerant of radishes. Both TDI and radishes contain allyl isothiocyanate and benzyl isothiocyanate, but other foods containing these same chemicals did not provoke symptoms. The authors were unable to speculate as to the possible mechanism for this cross-sensitivity. Indoor air contains organic compounds also found in foods, such as the fragrances limonene and pinene (see Table 4-2).

McGovern and associates (1981–82) have also written about chemical and food cross-sensitivity and noted that many foods contain phenolic derivatives. Chemically sensitive patients also frequently react to phenolic inhalants. The McGovern group attempted to desensitize patients to particular phenolics and noted very robust reactions to such challenges. Rea (1988a) reports food sensitivities in 80 percent of his patients with chemical sensitivities. Like airborne pollutants, foods contain a wide range of chemical constituents and are in intimate contact with the organism for long periods of time. The surface area of the gastrointestinal tract is enormous, and the chemical load, in terms of both quantity and diversity of exposure, is huge. From a developmental perspective, the contents of the gastrointestinal tract can be thought of not simply as part of the organism, but as "an insinuation of the environment into the body" (Angyal 1981).

Those IgE-mediated allergic reactions affecting the skin or lungs are more accessible for study than those affecting the gastrointestinal tract. The skin can be viewed directly, and devices are available for measuring changes in pulmonary function. Dean Metcalfe of the National Institutes of Health (1986) comments:

> The situation is much different when it comes to allergic diseases that involve the gastrointestinal tract. This system is relatively inaccessible and difficult to study and, thus far, less information has accumulated relative to allergic reactions in its tissues.

Yet, the potential for allergic reactions in the gastrointestinal tract is present: mast cells, the cells that release chemical mediators that result in an allergic reaction, are more densely packed in the intestinal tract ($20,000/mm^3$) than in the skin ($7,000/mm^3$), another organ considered rich in mast cells (Barrett 1984).

The food intolerances of patients with multiple chemical sensitivities may or may not be IgE-mediated or involve mast cell release of histamine or other mediators. In any case, the difficulties in studying adverse reactions to foods are the same. The inaccessibility of the gastrointestinal tract and its enormous chemical and antigenic contents greatly encumber study of chemical mediators or subtle pathophysiological alterations. Whatever the mechanism, conducting blinded food challenges is difficult to accomplish without altering the food in some respect. Dehydrated foods administered in opaque capsules may not provoke the same response as larger quantities of fresh foods. Some individuals may react to the capsules themselves or fail to react if food does not contact the oral mucosa.

Whether in reference to foods, drugs, or other chemicals, adaptation may occur, altering the organism's later responses to and tolerance for other substances. The mechanisms are unknown, but this does not preclude our recognition of or intervention in this problem. The use of an environmental unit may provide a way of unmasking or backing up the experience or, as Randolph (1976a) states, provide "the means of reverting many chronic illnesses of unknown cause to acute illness in which specific etiology is readily demonstrated."

Summary of Adaptation Hypotheses.   We acknowledge the complexity of the concept of adaptation. Here we summarize the salient points concerning this topic.

Symptoms of exposure to many chemicals, whether inhaled or ingested, appear to follow a biphasic pattern. Adaptation is characterized by acclimatization (habituation, tolerance) with repeated exposures that result in a masking of symptoms. Withdrawal occurs when exposure is discontinued. Once a person has adapted, then the experimental consequences are that further exposures have very little additional effect and therefore may not be observed. The observer may not be able to witness the stimulatory or reactive event because a kind of "saturation" effect has set in.

Adaptation and withdrawal occur for a wide variety of organic and inorganic substances in many physical forms, including various dusts and fumes, solvents, nitroglycerin, ozone, and foods.

An individual is exposed to a variety of substances at different times with varying frequency, duration, and intensity of exposure for each of these substances and with varying frequency and duration of reduction in or cessation of exposure for each substance. The individual may be in different stages (stimulatory or withdrawal) simultaneously for different substances. These stages may overlap (see Fig. 2-2) and interfere with attempts to observe cause-and-effect relationships.

Adaptation may mask some symptoms or effects while other physiological alterations may continue.

Comprehensive environmental control, that is, an environmental unit, may overcome the masking effect of adaptation and the problems of overlapping exposures that result in overlapping responses to multiple agents. The environmental unit may allow the investigator to back up or reverse the experience of adaptation and monitor toxicity in progress. The advantages dynamic toxicity of this nature may have over conventional methods for determining toxicity include facilitating detection of sublclinical, prepathological effects of chemicals and providing more than just a snapshot of an individual's response to substances. Removing the person from interacting, time-dependent stimuli in this way may allow the unraveling of multiple causes . The environmental unit may be an essential tool. Many carefully conducted studies of chemical effects that have had negative or equivocal outcomes may be flawed by their failure to take adaptive mechanisms into account. The consequences of such an oversight could be major

The Environmental Unit

Adaptation and the use of an environmental unit are complex topics that do not lend themselves to the short presentations typical of most scientific forums. Yet, physicians must understand adaptation if progress is to be made in this field. Some of the allergists we spoke with recognize the pivotal role adaptation may play. Prominent among them is John Selner, an allergist who has long advocated that allergists take a more active role in understanding patients with alleged chemical sensitivities and who described in detail the design and operation of an environmental unit (Selner and Staudenmayer 1985a). Selner visited Rea's unit in Dallas and collaborated with Ken Gerdes, an ecologist who trained with Randolph, to establish a unit in Denver at Presbyterian–St. Luke Hospital in 1979. This unit, which operated for several years before closing for reasons unrelated to its utility as a diagnostic tool, incorporated many if not most of the features of existing clinical ecology units. Rea and Randolph, who had their own units, both visited Selner's unit when it opened and admired the care that had been exercised in its construction. Without exception, all allergists with whom we spoke agreed that an environmental unit like Selner's was an important tool for properly evaluating patients with alleged low-level chemical sensitivities. Few, however, appreciate the degree to which Selner patterned his approach after that developed by the clinical ecologists.

The clinical ecologists' environmental units and Selner's unit shared many of the same design and operational parameters (Table 2-6).

We are unable to discern any major differences in these two approaches. Even though Selner's unit is no longer in operation, he continues to employ some of the same principles, such as housing patients

TABLE 2-6. Features of Environmental Units[a]

Characteristics/Practices	Allergists' Unit[b]	Clinical Ecologists' Units[c]
Construction using materials that do not off-gas (primarily glass, steel, ceramic; cotton bedding and clothing). Avoidance of synthetic materials. No perfumes, cosmetics, odorous cleaners/soaps, etc.	Yes	Yes
Air supply filtered; patients' rooms under positive pressure to reduce contamination from adjacent areas; airlocks	Yes	Yes
Patients' medications discontinued insofar as possible; gradual withdrawal from steroids, etc.	Yes	Yes
Patients fasted for 4 to 8 days to clear symptoms.	Yes, if symptoms do not clear after several days in unit	Yes, at time of admission to unit
Organic foods used for food testing; commercial foods tested also	Yes	Yes
Patients tested for acceptable water	Yes	Yes
Challenges performed using single foods and chemicals after period of avoidance (to eliminate masking)	Yes	Yes

[a] None of the units described in this table is currently in operation.

[b] Selner in Denver (Selner and Staudenmayer, 1985a).

[c] Randolph in Chicago and Rea in Dallas.

in a relatively clean environment to try to avoid chemical exposure prior to testing. In Selner's view, the fundamental concept is still valid. He states, as do Rea and Randolph, that the majority of patients can be worked up as outpatients. However, a small percentage of patients are difficult to evaluate without such a facility.

Studies from the ecologists' units leave much to be desired in terms of study design. Unfortunately, no studies were ever published from the allergists' unit in Denver. *Every* traditional allergist we interviewed recognized that removal from exposure prior to testing might be a critical factor in studying reactions to low levels of chemicals. They felt that reestablishment of a unit would be an important step in understanding the problems of individuals who believe they are sensitive to low levels of chemicals. In fact, some of the allergists offered examples for which removal from exposure for several days prior to testing would be important, such as exposure to western red cedar or cigarette smoke. They were not at all opposed to the concept of an environmental unit and were aware of the considerable expense involved in establishing a well-designed and well-run environmental unit.

Some allergists we interviewed felt ecologists should be involved in the design of a study unit and appropriate protocols because of their experience in this area and so as to avoid later criticism from the ecologists regarding the protocols that are used. Two of the traditional allergists we interviewed praised Rea's engineering skills in designing and operating his unit, one saying, "No one does it as well as Rea does." Rea has, in fact, stated his willingness to cooperate with any impartial venture to undertake studies using his facilities or to design a model research unit elsewhere.

Although the detailed description of an environmental unit is beyond the limits of this discussion, some of the essentials are noted here.

First, by employing construction materials, furnishings, and clothing that are less likely to off-gas, very low levels of volatile organic compounds (for example, from synthetics) can be maintained inside the unit. To create and operate a unit that is as free as possible from chemical pollution requires knowledge, precision, and vigilance while working with architects, ventilation engineers, contractors and their suppliers, nurses, dieticians, food and water suppliers, and maintenance and custodial staffs. Obviously, "this is no trifling undertaking" (Selner and Staudenmeyer 1985a). Three basic scientific approaches for studying a disease are clinicopathological studies, animal experiments, and epidemiological investigations. To these, Randolph (1965) has added a fourth tool, comprehensive environmental control. Animal models, clinicopathological studies, and epidemiological investigations have certain important limitations for studying the phenomenon of multiple chemical sensitivities. None is as sensitive to low-level exposures and effects as the use of an environmental unit in which all exposures are controlled simultaneously and the individual is challenged with single substances while in the deadapted state. A theoretical, graphical representation of an individual's responses to environmental incitants before entering an environmental unit, after entering the unit, and during challenges to single incitants appears in Figure 2-3.

Animal models are best used to study relatively high doses of chemicals that result in distinctive physical or biochemical *pathology* that can be monitored. First, an appropriate animal must be found. Next are concerns about extrapolations to humans. More importantly here, rats, mice, and other animals are unable to tell researchers if they have headaches, feel depressed or anxious, or are nauseated. Thus the subtle effects of low-level chemical exposure may be missed entirely.

Epidemiology may have some utility with regard to tight buildings or community exposures to a toxic material. If everyone in the population responds with the same symptoms to the same agents, the task is relatively easy. However, if some people have headaches, others have muscle spasms, and still others are less able to concentrate, the results blur and may wash out entirely; that is, no single symptom has a statistically significant prevalence over controls. Thus, for multiple chemical sensitivities with multiple triggers and multiple health effects, epidemiology may be an insensitive tool. Further, although epidemiology can point to *associations* between events, other kinds of studies are needed to establish cause-and-effect relationships. In the study of chemical sensitivity, identification of an unaffected control group presents further difficulties.

Clinicopathological studies rely upon the presence of some clinical sign (for example, tachycardia or decreased reflexes), laboratory measurement, or tissue pathology. For meaningful data in humans, large numbers of similarly exposed individuals with similar end-organ effects must be examined. Again, multiple chemical sensitivities may involve multiple triggers and multiple effects. To date, no single laboratory test is abnormal in most, much less all, who are affected. At some point in the future, such a test or marker may be discovered, but for now no mass applicable clinical, laboratory, or pathological findings are available. Further, subjective complaints of patients may be overlooked, particularly if they vary from one person to the next. Thus clinicopathological studies are not likely to be sensitive to the early effects of low-level exposures, that is, prior to end-organ damage.

What is needed is a sensitive tool that reliably detects symptoms of exposure to low levels of multiple chemicals in human beings, taking into account individual variability, a tool that will allow us to ascertain cause-and-effect relationships between exposures and symptoms. The environmental unit **could be** such a tool. Potentially, it may be the most useful of the four approaches for studying human response to environmental agents. For this reason, if for no other, the EPA and other governmental bodies concerned with regulating exposure to low levels of toxic environmental agents should take great interest in this approach. The individuals who might enter environmental units perhaps represent the most susceptible population. Their responses to chemical challenges while in a deadapted state in an environmental unit would further our understanding of low-level chemical sensitivity. Carefully designed and orchestrated studies with meticulous attention to the details of environmental control, as defined by those who have operated such units, are essential to resolving these issues to the satisfaction of all.

Graphical Representation of an Individual's Symptoms Before and After Entering an Environmental Unit

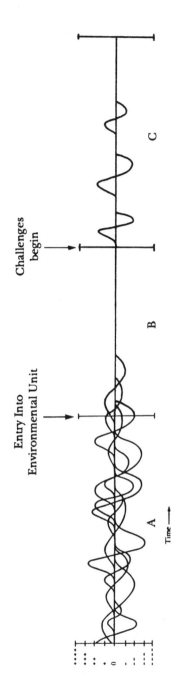

Figure 2-3. In time period A an individual is responding to multiple incitants encountered in normal daily living (chemicals and/or foods), with stimulatory and withdrawal effects that overlap in time. At any particular time, how the person feels is determined not only by ongoing exposures, but by previous exposures whose effects may still be waning. In time period B, the individual enters an environmentally controlled facility, fasting. With cessation of contributory exposures, withdrawal effects occur, for example, headache, fatigue, and myalgias. Symptoms continue for some time (typically 4 -7 days) until the individual reaches "0" baseline. In time period C, single challenges to suspected incitants are administered. Symptoms, often robust, develop soon after challenges, allowing patient and physician to begin to observe the relationship between exposures and symptoms for that individual.

CHAPTER 3

Origins of Multiple Chemical Sensitivity and Effects on Health

Offending Substances

This chapter addresses the origins of multiple chemical sensitivity, that is, the offending substances that may induce the illness, as well as those that trigger symptoms once the problem has begun. In Chapter 2, adaptation was discussed in relation to several different materials, including ozone, nitroglycerin, cotton dust, metal fumes, solvents, alcohol, and tobacco smoke. Clinical ecologists and their patients have noted adaptation to an enormous range of substances that can be categorized as outdoor air pollutants; indoor air pollutants, both domestic and workplace; food contaminants and additives; water contaminants and additives; and drugs and consumer products.

In preparing this book, we considered referencing representative articles from toxicology that would show that substances in the above categories may be toxic to animals or humans. However, an encyclopedic listing would have little point. Certainly toxic substances in the environment have adverse health consequences. The question is whether certain persons develop heightened reactivity to chemicals and foods, and if so, why?

John Selner, an allergist critical of clinical ecology yet who advocates the use of an environmental unit for diagnosing certain patients, studied these hyperreactive individuals but regrettably has published no studies of patients in his former environmental unit. His and others' criticisms and studies to disprove this field have not involved independent investigations in which food and chemical challenges on patients in a deadapted state were performed. Thus, Randolph's observations on adaptation have not yet been replicated, even though adaptation would seem an important hypothesis to test. Most ot the allergists' criticisms have been aimed at the efficacy of treatments, for example, provocation-neutralization, for chemically sensitive patients. These critiques of treatment modalitites and an absence of consistent laboratory abnormalities have been used as the basis for trying to disprove existence of the illness altogether.

Clinical ecologists, as well as some allergists (Selner 1988) with whom we spoke, invoke the concept of total body load or burden. To ecologists, this load is comprised of all incitants to which the body must respond (adapt) to maintain homeostasis. They may be chemical, biological (pollens, molds, bacteria, viruses), physical (heat, cold, radiation), or psychological. Notwithstanding its utility as a theoretical construct to help "explain" why this disorder occurs in a given individual, total load per se is not measurable. However, part of it can be quantified. For example, Laseter and co-workers (1983) measured levels of 16 chlorinated hydrocarbon pesticides in 200 chemically sensitive patients, 99 percent of whom had residues at or above 0.05 ppb in their blood, reflecting even higher tissue levels. The mean was 3.4 pesticides per patient. Volatile organic hydrocarbons (Rea 1987) and aliphatic hydrocarbon solvents (Pan et al. 1987–88) have also been measured in these patients, but their levels have not been compared with those of individuals who do not have such symptoms. Nevertheless, Rea and others feel that these substances are not normal constituents of the body and therefore represent a substantial burden for the individual. However, even if *no* differences in levels existed between chemically sensitive patients and so-called normals, these compounds still could be a source of their illness because chemically sensitive patients may be a subgroup of the population that is more susceptible to the effects of these chemicals. In addition, what may be most relevant is their *past* exposure that may have caused them to become sensitized in the first place.

Some authors have attempted to distinguish between those chemical exposures associated with the *onset* of multiple chemical sensitivity syndrome and those associated with *recurrence* of symptoms, that is, act as triggers once the syndrome has developed. Cone and associates (1987) studied workers with multiple chemical sensitivities, 11 of whom reported that solvent exposures of various types had caused their problem; three pointed to pesticide exposures; one, hydrogen sulfide; one, copy machines; one, new materials including carpets. Once the syndrome had developed, triggers for recurrence of symptoms in these same patients were far more diverse and included such common exposures as tobacco smoke, perfume, scented soap, car exhaust, copiers, gas stoves, tar, smog, newspapers, new clothing in stores, leather, printed books, office buildings, and glues.

In Terr's (1986) review of 50 cases seen by clinical ecologists, 43 cases of which were referred to him by workers' compensation carriers for independent evaluation, the patients also attributed their illness to a wide array of exposures: 16 complained of acute exposure to a chemical, three from pesticides, two from phenol; 34 patients felt their illness resulted from chronic exposures, six from unspecified chemicals in their homes, four from office machines, three from organic solvents, three from smoke, three from foods, two from formaldehyde, two from the hospital environment, and two from airplanes. These reports reflect fairly well the variety of exposures that clinical ecologists allege precede their patients' illness.

Subsequently Terr (1989a) compiled findings from 40 of these 50 cases plus an additional 50 cases; all patients had previously seen an ecologist and had applied for workers' compensation. Of these 90 patients, 28 had symptoms corresponding to a single organ system and 62 had multisystem polysymptomatic complaints. Table 2-3 summarizes the exposures these patients felt had caused their condition: 83 identified one or more (up to six) causative agents. Exposure durations ranged from a few seconds to 20 years. Table 2-4 lists their occupations: 19 were engaged in office work, 13 in transportation, 12 in electronics manufacturing, 11 in medicine or social work, eight in education, eight in other manufacturing, and the remainder distributed among a variety of other occupations.

It is conceivable that chemical sensitivity involves a two-step process: Certain exposures may induce the illness, whereas others may simply trigger symptoms once the syndrome has developed. We next discuss in more detail the range and nature of exposures that are thought to contribute to this problem and explore the five subgroups of exposures mentioned at the beginning of this chapter.

Health effects data on chemicals are notoriously inadequate. A 1984 study by the National Research Council attempted to assess the testing needs for various industrial and consumer chemicals (National Research Council 1984). Figure 3-1 shows existing needs for health hazard assessment and toxicity data. No toxicity data or minimal data are available for 66 percent of pesticides and their supposedly inert ingredients, 84 percent of cosmetic ingredients, 64 percent of drugs, 81 percent of food additives, and 88 to 90 percent of chemicals in commerce.

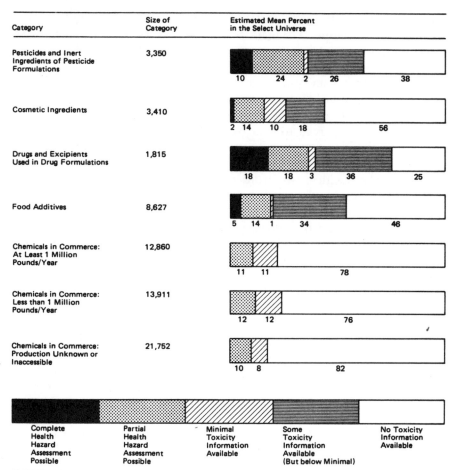

Category	Size of Category	Estimated Mean Percent in the Select Universe
Pesticides and Inert Ingredients of Pesticide Formulations	3,350	10 24 2 26 38
Cosmetic Ingredients	3,410	2 14 10 18 56
Drugs and Excipients Used in Drug Formulations	1,815	18 18 3 36 25
Food Additives	8,627	5 14 1 34 46
Chemicals in Commerce: At Least 1 Million Pounds/Year	12,860	11 11 78
Chemicals in Commerce: Less than 1 Million Pounds/Year	13,911	12 12 76
Chemicals in Commerce: Production Unknown or Inaccessible	21,752	10 8 82

Complete Health Hazard Assessment Possible	Partial Health Hazard Assessment Possible	Minimal Toxicity Information Available	Some Toxicity Information Available (But below Minimal)	No Toxicity Information Available

FIGURE 3-1. *Ability to conduct health-hazard assessment of substances in seven categories of a select universe of chemicals.*
Source: National Research Council 1984.

Thus, scientific data concerning health effects of the vast majority of chemicals are woefully lacking. Chemically sensitive patients may fill in the gaps long before toxicologists do.

Outdoor Air Pollutants

Among the most hazardous exposures for patients seem to be pesticides sprayed either outdoors or indoors. Alone, pesticides have accounted for some of the most advanced and persistent cases of chemical sensitivity known to clinical ecologists. As early as 1966, occupational health practitioners observed that certain persons who had "recovered" from acute organophosphate pesticide poisoning experienced protracted symptoms of nausea, headache, irritability, insomnia, inability to concentrate, blurred vision, or shakiness (Tabershaw and Cooper 1966). Twenty of 114 individuals stated they could no longer tolerate smelling or contact with pesticides. Depression and schizophrenia occurred in others (Gershon and Shaw 1961). Neuropsychiatric, cardiopulmonary, and gastrointestinal symptoms may persist long after exposure to organophosphate insecticides (Namba et al. 1971), which are widely used by exterminators indoors and out-of-doors. Other outdoor exposures presenting problems for the chemically susceptible patient include vapors from solvents and fuels, combustion products, tar fumes, paint vapors, diesel and auto exhaust, and industrial air pollution (Randolph 1962).

The adverse effects of air pollution upon individuals with respiratory or cardiac compromise are widely acknowledged. Less well known, but increasingly studied, have been associations between outdoor air pollutant levels and psychiatric emergency room visits (Briere et al. 1983; Strahilevitz et al. 1979), psychiatric hospital admissions (Strahilevitz et al. 1979), family disturbances (Rotton and Frey 1985), and anxiety symptoms (Evans et al. 1988).

Randolph described a woman who became ill each time she journeyed through the industrial pollution of northwestern Indiana and the south side of Chicago (Randolph 1987, pp. 73–76). Other patients note difficulty in any large metropolis, in the vicinity of airports, at bus or train stations, or in heavy traffic.

Diesel exhaust is a particular problem for many patients. In an EPA review of the toxicology of diesel exhaust, Nelson projected, "I think we can conclude quite straightforwardly that a major increase in the Diesel fleet is not going to produce a disastrous epidemic of lung cancer," but "risk assessment should be the ultimate goal and should be given the highest priority" (Nelson 1982). Many chemically sensitive patients experience severe symptoms with exposure to diesel exhaust. Interestingly, a Japanese study suggests that the striking increase in allergic rhinitis triggered by pollens that has occurred in that country over the past 30 years may be in part the result of lenient regulation of diesel exhaust and increased numbers of diesel vehicles (Muranaka et al. 1986). The authors note that the Japanese cedar, a tree indigenous to Japan for at least a million years, was never known to cause allergic rhinitis until 1964; and that before 1950 allergic rhinitis was virtually unknown in their country, although even then it had been recognized among Japanese living in the United States. Muranaka points to diesel exhaust as a possible cause for Japan's increasing allergic rhinitis.

In guinea pigs, short-term exposure to the ubiquitous air pollutant sulfur dioxide (SO_2), even at levels below national ambient air quality standards, augments subsequent allergic sensitization of the airways (Riedel 1988). Under the microscope, the bronchi (large airways) in SO_2-exposed guinea pigs appear inflamed and thus may be more permeable, facilitating access of antigens to the immune system. When provocation with inhaled antigen (ovalbumin) is performed repeatedly over a 3-week period, most of the SO_2-exposed animals show maximal bronchial reactions during the first few challenges. Continued provocation leads to a decrease in obstructive reactions that the authors describe as "allergen tachyphylaxis" but that might also fit the model of adaptation.

Chemical waste disposal sites may contaminate the air and groundwater of nearby communities. David Ozonoff of the Boston University School of Public Health and his co-workers (1987) surveyed households surrounding an odorous chemical waste disposal site and found that exposed individuals more often complained of respiratory symptoms (wheezing, shortness of breath, chest discomfort, persistent colds, coughs) and constitutional symptoms (chronic fatigue, bowel dysfunction, and irregular heartbeat) than did controls. Levels of air contaminants that were detected were exceedingly low and led the authors to conclude that the general population may react to chemicals at concentrations much lower than previously thought. Most studies of populations near hazardous waste facilities have focused on serious but low-prevalence diseases such as cancer. In small populations, such outcomes are difficult to measure because of low statistical power. The authors suggest that future investigations should concentrate instead upon common medical complaints: "Not only are such outcomes more amenable to study because of their higher prevalence, they may have considerable importance because of their impact on the efficiency, well-being, comfort, and productivity of a community."

As is discussed in the following section, indoor air pollution rather than outdoor air pollution accounts for the greatest number of and most intense exposures (Nero 1988). Most people spend the majority of their time indoors, either at work or home. Moreover, the levels of exposure to many contaminants, particularly volatile organic compounds (many of which are uncharacterized and whose health effects are unknown) are much higher indoors than out-of-doors.

Indoor Air Pollutants, Domestic and Workplace

The scope of indoor air pollutants has been reviewed by others (Spengler and Sexton 1983b; Nero 1988; Cone and Hodgson 1989). John Spengler of the Harvard School of Public Health, an authority on indoor air, predicts that the problem of buildings with unhealthy air is likely to continue for years because another generation of "pathologic" buildings is already on the drawing boards (Spengler 1989). He describes the "space flu" experienced by astronauts before NASA recognized that construction materials and supplies off-gassing inside a tightly sealed spacecraft were the source of the illness. Subsequently, NASA has compiled a detailed inventory of all materials used in their vehicles and the types and amounts of chemicals they release into the air and has designed spacecrafts to minimize exposures.

The range of indoor air pollutants affecting industrial workers is enormous. Seemingly, almost any process involving chemicals appears to have the potential for initiating chemical hyperreactivity via long- or short-term exposure. Two general types of exposures seem particularly apt to initiate hypersusceptibility:

1. A massive, overwhelming exposure, such as a chemical spill, a fire involving synthetic materials, pesticide spraying, or working with chemicals in a confined, unventilated space.

2. Repeated, low-level exposure to a complex array of synthetic organic compounds, as occurs with combustion products (such as diesel exhaust), tight buildings, and soldering (Miller 1979).

Gas chromatographic analysis of air samples from problem buildings or homes typically reveals the presence of multiple spiked peaks, each representing a particular organic compound (Fig. 3-2). Additional sampling and analytical approaches are needed to measure oxides of nitrogen from gas combustion, ozone, pesticide residues, and other air contaminants that may be present in the same environment.

At home, troublesome exposures for the chemically sensitive patient include the gas stove, one of the most commonly identified triggers of symptoms in these patients; combustion products from gas- or oil-fired furnaces and space heaters, water heaters, and central air heating systems; sponge rubber bedding, padding, and upholstery; plastics (especially pliable odorous plastics such as shower curtains); insecticides; perfumes; paints and decorating materials; fireplaces; cleaning agents; disinfectants; deodorizers; mothballs; cedar closets; newsprint and other printed materials; fabrics in clothing, bedding, and window coverings, especially synthetics or coated fabrics; particleboard; gasoline vapors from attached garages; and carpeting and carpet padding. Disinfectant liquids and sprays containing phenolics frequently provoke symptoms in these patients. Interestingly, researchers first became concerned about orthophenyl phenol when they noticed that mice housed in cages washed with this common institutional and household disinfectant showed markedly depressed immune responses after 4 to 6 weeks of exposure (La Via 1979).

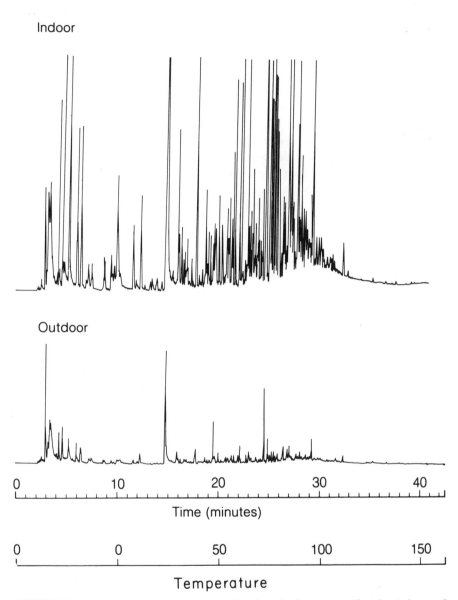

Indoor

Outdoor

Time (minutes)

Temperature

FIGURE 3-2. *A comparison of gas chromatographs of equal volume air samples taken indoors and outdoors near a complaint office building.*
Source: Miksch, R. R., Hollowell, C. D., Schmidt, H. E. "Trace Organic Chemical Contaminants in Office Spaces," Environ Int *8:129–138, 1982. Courtesy of Lawrence Berkeley Laboratory, University of California.*

The Environmental Protection Agency recently conducted air sampling for pesticides inside homes in Jacksonville, Florida, and Springfield and Chicopee, Massachusetts (Immerman 1990). (See Fig. 1-7). Analysis revealed a profile of multiple agents that had been applied over the life of each home. Pesticides applied years before and subsequently banned could be detected. Approximately eight different pesticides were detected in the average home in Florida, compared to four in Massachusetts (out of a total of 32 pesticides for which testing was done). Patients with chemical sensitivities sometimes associate onset of their illness with a particular move, and the potential role of previously applied, long-lived chemicals merits thoughtful scientific exploration.

Several guides for constructing homes from "safer" materials that are less toxic and/or do not off-gas have been written (Rousseau et al. 1988; Good and Dadd 1988; Zamm and Gannon 1980). Urea formaldehyde foam insulation, which may have provoked this illness in many in the past, has ceased being used by insulators since a flurry of successful lawsuits. As part of its research and information mandate under Title IV of the Superfund Amendments and Reauthorization Act of 1986, the EPA Indoor Air Division is currently developing several guidance documents on designing and operating buildings to ensure indoor air quality. These documents address the design and construction of residential and public and commercial buildings, the operation and maintenance of public and commercial buildings, and indoor air quality management in schools.

Mobile homes and automobile interiors present their own special problems. Indoor air pollutants in other settings may present problems: shopping malls, perfume counters, detergent and insecticide aisles, fabric stores, dry cleaners, deodorizers and hairspray in public rest rooms, tobacco smoke, incense, Sterno used in buffets, gas cooking combustion products in restaurants, and perfume, cologne, or mothball odors on garments worn in theaters, churches, and public transport commonly cause difficulty for these patients. "Odors" of virtually any desription, especially petrochemical odors but also "natural" odors from cedar or pine terpenes or cooking foods, may provoke symptoms; the presence of an odor implies that the substance in question has a vapor pressure and that molecules of it are present in the air. The subject of odors and their role in this syndrome is discussed in Chapter 4.

Historical Notes.   Randolph first discussed the topic of indoor air pollution in a series of articles published in 1954 and subsequently in *Human Ecology and Susceptibility to the Chemical Environment* in 1962. That same year, President Kennedy called the first national conference on air pollution in Washington, D.C. It was a 3-day program with only an hour and a half at the end for open discussion. During the discussion, Randolph remarked that in 3 days of presentations not a single reference had been made to *indoor* air pollution. In his clinical experience, he said, indoor air pollution was 8 to 10 times more important as a source of illness in susceptible individuals than outdoor air pollution. Whereas outdoor air pollution tended to be intermittent and variable, indoor air pollution was much more constant. Further, individuals spend the majority of their time indoors. He also noted that more than 800 gas stoves had been removed from the homes of his highly susceptible patients.

Twenty years later, pollution from the same sources Randolph had identified as triggers of his patients' symptoms was documented by advanced and sensitive analytical techniques such as gas chromatography with mass spectrophotometry, which was not available at the time of Randolph's original writings. Between 1979 and 1985, the EPA undertook an extensive study of exposures to volatile organic compounds of 400 residents in three states (Wallace 1987). The TEAM study (total exposure assessment methodology) employed state-of-the-art monitoring and analytical methods. Each subject wore a personal air sampler for 24 hours and provided a breath sample at the end of the day. Personal exposures were consistently greater than outdoor levels, sometimes by factors of 10 or more (closely approximating Randolph's estimates 20 years earlier), implying important indoor sources of exposure. Smoking, visiting the dry cleaner or gas station, and certain occupations resulted in very elevated exposures. Breath levels were 30 to 40 percent of personal air concentrations for 9 of 11 compounds but ranged as high as 75 to 80 percent for benzene (from gasoline) and 90 percent for tetrachloroethylene (Wallace et al. 1985). Summarizing data from nine separate studies involving more than 1,000 homes, Wallace reported agreement on these points:

1. Essentially every one of the 40 or so organics studied has higher indoor levels than outdoor.
2. Sources are numerous, including building materials, furnishings, dry-cleaned clothes, cigarettes, gasoline, cleansers, moth crystals, hot showers, printed material, etc.
3. Ranges of concentrations are great, often 2 or more orders of magnitude.

Clearly, exposures in most indoor situations occur at levels well below current OSHA or EPA standards. At a given moment, several hundred different chemicals may be present in air samples from a home or office. One question that arises is whether the summation of all of these chemicals' effects could be responsible for symptoms, even though no single constituent accounts for them. To this end, Molhave (1986) of Denmark exposed 62 individuals to a mixture of 22 volatile organic compounds (VOCs) that commonly occur as indoor air pollutants. Three concentrations of total pollutants were used: 0 mg/m^3 (control), 5 mg/m^3, and 25 mg/m^3 of the same mixture of 22 compounds. Using "healthy" subjects (both male and female) who had previously complained about symptoms of sick building syndrome, Molhave exposed them to each concentration for 2.75-hour periods. As the air concentration increased, complaints of nasal and throat irritation and inability to concentrate (measured by digit span memory performance) rose. Thus, as the dose increased, these more "susceptible" individuals who otherwise appeared healthy were significantly affected by the indoor air pollutants, to the point of having difficulty with tasks requiring concentration.

In a follow-up study, undertaken to confirm and extend the 1986 Molhave study, Otto, Molhave, and co-workers (1989) exposed 66 normal, healthy males (with no history of chemical sensitivity) for 2.75 hours to a complex VOC mixture at 0 and 25 mg/m^3. The study confirmed perceptions of odor unpleasantness found in the 1986 study. However, VOC exposure did not affect performance on any behavioral tests. Certainly, the 2.75-hour exposure time used in both studies does not compare to the day in, day out exposures of occupants of tight buildings. Nevertheless, comparison of the two studies suggests differences in central nervous system effects between healthy individuals and those who have complained of indoor air problems previously. Unfortunately, because of the irritant effects from exposure to higher levels of VOCs, blinding is exceedingly difficult to achieve in the design of such studies.

Other Scandinavian researchers have found total volatile organic compound concentrations in homes with complaints by occupants to average 1.3 mg/m^3 (range 0.092 to 13 mg/m^3), whereas the concentrations in houses where there were no complaints averaged 0.36 mg/m^3 (range 0.02 to 1.7 mg/m^3) (Molhave 1986–87). Thus, levels of volatile organic compounds were generally higher in problem houses.

Studying the white-collar work environment, Robertson et al. (1985) compared health problems in two office buildings, one fully air-conditioned and the other naturally ventilated. Sickness was significantly increased in the air-conditioned building versus the naturally ventilated building, particularly rhinitis (28 percent versus 5 percent), nasal blockage and dry throat (35 percent versus 9 percent), lethargy (36 percent versus 13 percent), and headache (31 percent versus 15 percent). That temperature, humidity, air velocity, and other such factors did not differ between the two buildings suggests that the sickness was caused by indoor air pollutants. Similarly, Finnegan and co-workers (1984) found significant excesses of eye, nose, and mucous membrane symptoms, as well as lethargy, dry skin, and headaches among workers in air-conditioned versus naturally ventilated offices.

An unanticipated and unwelcome opportunity for the EPA to study the effects of indoor air pollution firsthand arose when 27,000 square yards of new carpeting were installed in the agency's headquarters in Washington, D.C., in 1987 and 1988 (Hirzy and Morison 1989a, 1989b). An estimated 124 of 2,000 employees exposed to volatile off-gassing from the carpet became ill, exhibiting symptoms ranging from eye, nose, and throat irritation and breathing problems to nausea, headache, dizziness, difficulty in thinking, fatigue, and increased susceptibility to many exposures formerly tolerated. At least two employees quit their jobs as a result of illness. Seventeen were unable to work in their assigned spaces. Some now work at home or in other locations. Eight report new sensitivities to common substances, including perfumes, auto exhaust, and tobacco smoke. Symptoms of the 20 or so most severely affected individuals appear identical to those of patients seen by clinical ecologists. Agency scientists in the employee's union who analyzed air samples felt the culprit might be 4-phenylcyclohexene (4-PC), which is used to bind carpet fabric to its backing. Estimates of the exposures that initiated illness in the susceptible subgroup range from 5 to 15 ppb of 4-PC (Hirzy and Morison 1989b). These same persons, now "sensitized," experience symptoms upon reexposure to less than 1 ppb of the substance; symptoms include respiratory difficulty, dizziness, "spacey" feelings, and general malaise. The EPA problem lends further credence to Randolph's and other clinical ecologists' observations with respect to: (1) diverse symptoms occurring in different individuals even with the same exposure, (2) "spreading" of sensitivities to other low-level chemical exposures and to foods that formerly had been tolerated, and (3) adaptation, that is, the less severely affected employees noted improvement in symptoms while away from work with marked increase upon return and gradual subsidence during the workweek as tolerance developed (Hirzy 1989).

Foods, Food Additives, and Contaminants

Rea (1988a) estimates that food sensitivity occurs in about 80 percent of his patients with chemical sensitivities. Ecologists observe that excessive chemical exposure may result in loss of tolerance to foods, sometimes to every food in the diet, and that removing the individual from such exposures and rotating foods so that no food is eaten more than once every 4 days may restore dietary tolerance. Pesticide residues, can linings (the gold-brown lining of cans may contain a phenolic resin), fumigants, fungicides, sulfur treatment, artificial colors, sweeteners, preservatives, ripening procedures (such as ethylene gas), protective waxes, and packaging materials, especially plastics, may trigger symptoms in patients. When patients are challenged with foods in an environmental unit, at first they are given chemically less contaminated foods such as organic meats and produce wherever possible. Once a variety of "safe" foods has been determined and prior to discharge from the unit, patients may be given several consecutive meals of commercial preparations of their safe foods. These meals might include commercial apples that have been sprayed (consider the recent concern over spraying apples with Alar, causing possible long-range effects in children who consume these apples or apple juice), canned foods, and nonorganic meats. After 2 days of such feedings, many patients reportedly experience fatigue, headache, myalgia, arthralgia, arthritis, depression, and other muscular, skeletal, and/or neurological symptoms (Randolph 1987).

Water Contaminants and Additives

According to Rea (1988a) as many as 90 percent of his patients with chemical sensitivities may have reactions to contaminants in drinking water. While fasting in an environmental unit, patients test waters from a variety of sources including tap water, specially distilled or filtered water, and various spring or well waters until they find one that does not evoke symptoms. Drinking water may be contaminated by leaching of chemicals from plastic storage containers, rubber hoses or connectors in distilling apparatus, or plastic or rubber fittings in drinking water dispensers. Uncontaminated well or spring water in glass bottles may be preferable for particularly sensitive individuals.

Chemical contamination of groundwater is a growing national concern. Aldicarb, a carbamate insecticide and nematocide used extensively since the 1960s, was first noted as a groundwater contaminant in the late 1970s, when more than 1,100 wells in New York's Suffolk County, a potato-farming region on Long Island, tested positive for aldicarb (levels greater than 7 ppb). Since that time, aldicarb has been found in groundwater in Maine, Florida, California, Arizona, North Carolina, Virginia, and Wisconsin. In Wisconsin, 23 apparently healthy women who consumed groundwater with detectable aldicarb were found to have altered T-cell subsets with a decreased $T_4:T_8$ ratio of 1.88 versus 2.54 in an unexposed control group ($p < 0.05$) (Fiore et al. 1986). Unlike AIDS, in which the $T_4:T_8$ ratio is decreased primarily because T_4 (helper) cells are destroyed by the virus, these women had an increase in T_8 (suppressor) cells. In addition, lymphocyte proliferation in response to *Candida* allergen was increased ($p < 0.02$) versus controls. Likewise, among residents of Woburn, Massachusetts, who drank water that had been contaminated with industrial solvents, excess leukemias (12 versus 5.3 expected), immunological abnormalities including decreased T-cell ratios (p <0.01), increased autoantibodies and infections, and neurological, cardiac, and skin abnormalities were noted (Byers et al. 1988). (See also Chapter 4.)

Ingestion is not the sole route of exposure to contaminants in water. Brown and associates (1984) reported that skin absorption (for example, from bathing or showering) may be a significant portal of entry for water contaminants accounting for 29 to 91 percent (average 64 percent) of the total daily dose of these substances. Aside from skin contact, showering volatilizes contaminants in water and leads to inhalation of chlorine, chloroform, and organic compounds (Bailey and Vanderslice 1987; Foster and Chrostowski 1987). Water contaminated with organic material and subsequently chlorinated contains chlorinated hydrocarbons that are potentially carcinogenic. Interestingly, chemically sensitive individuals frequently note symptoms while bathing or showering, and some claim they must use specially filtered water or at least water treated to remove the chlorine.

Drugs and Consumer Products

Physicians recognize that a person who has an adverse reaction to one drug is more likely to react to other drugs. The allergist Sullivan (1989) reported that individuals who experienced an adverse reaction to penicillin are much more likely to react adversely to other drugs, in particular, other antibiotics. Interestingly, he calls this phenomenon, which occurs in a very small percentage of the population, the "multiple drug allergy syndrome." The mechanism is unclear but he postulates it may be related to faulty regulation of antihapten immune responses. Meggs (1989a) compiled a list of symptoms that have been reported for seven well-known pharmaceuticals (indomethacin, propranolol, azatadine, pseudoephedrine, captopril, diazepam, and reserpine); these symptoms reproduced about 80 percent of the symptoms and complaints Terr (1989a) reported in patients exposed to various organic chemicals. Meggs comments, "Perhaps there is a similarity between adverse reactions to pharmaceuticals and volatile organic compounds found in the workplace. Again we are dealing with low molecular weight carbon-based compounds of similar structure in the two cases."

Randolph (1962, pp. 85–87) surveyed one series of 80 and another series of 250 of his chemically sensitive patients who had "known" reactions to some facet of their chemical environment and found that an extraordinarily high percentage had reacted adversely to one or more medications. One quarter to one half claimed to have reacted to aspirin, barbiturates, or sulfonamides. According to Randolph, because of this proneness to drug reactions and because many physicians do not understand this problem, many individuals with chemical sensitivities are reluctant to seek health care. Thus there seems to be an important overlap between individuals who react badly to medications and chemically sensitive patients. Investigating whether a disproportionate number of the idiosyncratic reactions listed in the *Physicians' Desk Reference* occur in the same subgroup of patients would be worthwhile. The psychiatrist Schottenfeld (1987) confirms that many individuals with multiple chemical sensitivities appear unusually sensitive to the anti cholinergic and sedative effects of tricyclic antidepressants.

Drugs, of course, contain much more than active ingredients. They also contain excipients (for example, cornstarch or lactose in tablets), diluents, coloring agents, flavorings, various coatings, and/or preservatives (as in allergy shots, which often contain about 0.4 percent phenol). Mineral oils, petroleum jelly, ointment, lotions, laxatives, synthetic vitamins, and adhesive tape cause problems for many patients. Most cosmetics, scented soaps, shampoos, hand lotions, personal hygiene products, perfumes, colognes, deodorants, hairsprays, hair dyes, mouthwashes, denture adhesives, and bath salts and oils have been reported to provoke reactions in individual patients. Many patients do better by substituting "natural" products for petrochemical ones (Ziem 1989).

In addition, permanent press finishes (especially during ironing); synthetic textiles; clothes that have been dry-cleaned; residues of detergents and fabric softeners; electric blankets (the plastic coatings over the wires off-gas when heated); waterbeds; mattresses treated with flame retardants; felt-tip pens; odorous books, magazines, and newsprint; polishes, cleaners, and bleaches; and chlorinated swimming pools and even bath and shower water have also been associated with intolerance (Randolph 1962, pp. 112–114).

The very ill patient may be sensitive to most if not all of these substances and products and has difficulty avoiding them and finding suitable substitutes. Mail-order services, often begun by patients, have developed to help sensitive individuals find products that are better tolerated. Exposures may be very subtle. For example, individuals may find themselves irritable or anxious when talking on the telephone, but if they substitute Bakelite phones for their new colored plastic ones or use speakerphones instead, their problem resolves (Randolph 1962). Clothing that was stored in particleboard drawers may emit formaldehyde and trigger symptoms. Synthetic fabrics have been implicated in elevated blood pressure, increased heart rate, arrhythmias, and angina

(Seyal et al. 1986a–d). Acrylic dentures may provoke headache, joint pain, fatigue, and rashes (Kroker et al. 1982).

The process of discovering the limits of one's tolerance may be long and tedious, with many setbacks. The setbacks can be so painful and disabling that patients go to great lengths to educate themselves about chemicals and avoid them. Very sensitive patients may react adversely to contact lenses, dental materials, medical implants or prostheses, local anesthetics, plasticizers leaching from plastic IV or oxygen lines, lubricating jelly applied during an examination, or alcohol evaporating on the skin when blood is drawn. Such patients view any encounter with an unknowing or disbelieving dentist or physician with great trepidation. Radio-contrast dyes may be of special concern. If surgery is planned, patients may inquire what intravenous solutions will be used (D_5 is 5 percent dextrose and thus contains corn sugar; corn is the most common food that provokes symptoms in these patients [Randolph and Moss 1980, p. 109]), what anesthetic drugs will be used, and the like, so as to prepare themselves and their doctors for any adverse reaction and attempt to avert it. Many practitioners find such inquiry intimidating or view the patient as demanding or hypochondriacal, when in fact the patient, in need of an operation or special procedure, only wishes to avoid an adverse reaction. Practitioners need to understand these patients' concerns and realize that the patients' fears may be well founded in prior experiences with very painful or embarrassing reactions. When they must place themselves in the hands of the medical establishment, chemically sensitive patients feel a lack of control and a vulnerability most would not understand.

Health Effects

According to the clinical ecologist, the symptoms and diseases caused by food and chemical exposures involve any and every system of the body and are so diverse that many traditional practitioners find them unbelievable. Some of the physicians we interviewed recalled being told as medical students that the more symptoms a patient complained of, the less validity any of them had. Clearly, such a belief by physicians could pose an obstacle in that the average patient with food and chemical sensitivities who enters an environmental unit has five symptoms, many of them neurological (Johnson and Rea 1989).

To many nonecologists, a troublesome aspect of the provocative food and chemical challenges performed by clinical ecologists has been the differences seen in symptoms on challenge versus those that were part of the patient's chief complaint at presentation. In his critique of 50 patients who previously had been seen by clinical ecologists, Terr (1986), an allergist, noted that 30 of the patients (60 percent) developed one or more *new* symptoms during their diagnostic and therapeutic experience with the clinical ecologist. Of these, the most frequent were headache (30 percent), fatigue (23 percent), confusion or loss of memory (20 percent), swelling (20 percent), dizziness (17 percent), depression (17 percent), nausea (17 percent), and rash, drowsiness, anxiety, and abdominal pain (13 percent). Forty-three of Terr's 50 patients were referred for workers' compensation evaluation and thus represent the "worst" cases. In comparison, less than 5 percent of the patients seen by Randolph and about 20 percent of those seen by Rea (who sees sicker patients referred by other ecologists) apply for disability.

In a more recent paper, Terr (1989a) compiled data from 40 of his original 50 patients plus 50 others claiming disability because of chemical sensitivities. Patients' symptoms were again diverse: 28 had symptoms referable to a single organ system, whereas 62 had "multisystem, polysymptomatology." After diagnosis of environmental illness by ecologists, 75 of these 90 workers reported one or more new triggers for their symptoms, including foods. These triggers were associated with one or more *new symptoms* in 34 patients.

The frequent emergence of new symptoms during deadaptation and reexposure is well known to clinical ecologists. Unfortunately, Terr does not offer any of the patients' commentary about their illness. However, 62 percent had a long history of multiple symptoms involving many systems and parts of the body and had been examined, tested, and treated unsuccessfully for years by many physicians prior to seeing a clinical ecologist. Perhaps some of their new symptoms did occur in the past but were transient in nature and forgotten. Perhaps adaptation masked certain symptoms. To the clinical ecologist, patients with very advanced environmental illness are manifesting the most extreme, overlapping stimulatory and withdrawal reactions to multiple substances. Chronic disability may ensue. However, the patient who is withdrawn from inciting chemical exposures and placed on a "safe" diet may be able to reverse the experience and begin to associate cause and effect. Specific symptoms can then be attributed to identifiable chemicals or foods in a reproducible way. Following deadaptation, symptoms that have not been experienced for decades may be manifested; that is, unmasking takes place. As long as multiple exposures causing multiple effects are overlapping, symptoms are masked and the person may experience chronic disability or ultimately end organ failure of some type.

The acute symptoms experienced by a patient when a clinical challenge is performed must be differentiated (Table 3-1) from the chronic disease states that are purported to result from chronic exposure to

TABLE 3-1. Possible Acute Reactions to Incitants during Provocation

Nasal	Throat, mouth	Ears	Lungs, heart, blood vessels	Joints	Muscles
Urge to sneeze	Itching, sore, tight, swollen	Itching	Coughing	Ache, pain	Tight, stiff
Itching, rubbing	Dysphagia, difficulty in swallowing, choking	Full, blocked	Sneezing	Stiff	Aches, soreness, pain
Obstruction		Erythema of pinna (reddening)	Reduced air flow	Swelling	Neck
Discharge	Weak voice, hoarse	Tinnitus (ringing in ears)	Retracting, shortnesss of breath	Erythema, warmth, redness	Upper, lower back
Postnasal drip	Salivation, mucus	Earache	Heavy, tight chest		Upper, lower extremities
Sinus discomfort	Bad or metallic taste	Hearing loss	Not enough air		
Stuffy feeling		Hyperacusis (abnormal sensitivity to sound)	Hyperventilation, rapid breathing		
			Chest pain		
			Tachycardia (rapid pulse)		
			Palpitations (rapid, violent or throbbing pulses; extra or skipped beats)		
			Blood vessels—spontaneous bruising and petechiae, cold sensitivity, swelling, acneform lesions		

Skin	Eyes	Vision	Cerebral, head	Genitourinary	Gastrointestinal
Itching, local or general	Itching, burning, pain	Blurring	Headache, mild–moderate; migraine	Voided, mild urge	Nausea
Scratching	Lacrimation (tearing)	Acuity decreased	Ache, pressure; tight, exploding feelings	Frequency in voiding	Belching
Moist, sweating	Injected light sensitive	Spots, flashes	Throbbing, stabbing	Urgency, pressure	Full, bloated
Flushing, hives	Sensitivity (allergic) shiners	Darker, vision loss	Fainting	Dysuria (painful or difficult urination)	Vomiting
Pallor (white or ghostly)	Feel heavy	Photophobia (brighter)	Depression	Genital itch	Pressure, pain, cramps
		Diplopia (double vision)	Mood swings	Vaginal discharge	Flatus, rumbling, gas
		Dyslexia–difficulty reading, transposition of letters; letters or words becoming small or large; words moving around	Hallucinations	Yeast infection	Diarrhea
			Hyperactivity		Gallbladder symptoms
			Irritability		Hunger, thirst
			Fatigue		Hyperacidity
			Apathy		
			Confusion		
			Lethargy		
			Blackouts		
			Insomnia		
			Somnolence		

Source: Rea, W., *Outpatient Information Manual* (1984a; 1988 revision), Environmental Health Center, Dallas.

incompatible foods and chemicals. The latter, according to clinical ecologists, include a wide range of diseases and disorders. Traditional practitioners consider many of these disorders idiopathic or essential (as in "essential hypertension") or give them names that are descriptive (as "asthma" or "urticaria") and are not revealing about possible causes. Clinical ecologists claim that many of these conditions are caused by environmental (food or chemical) incitants.

Perhaps the definitive test for chemical sensitivity would be to have the patient fast in an environmental unit. The resolution of chronic, debilitating symptoms then might suggest an environmental cause. Proof of environmental causation involves rechallenge with single foods and chemicals while noting the effects. If an effect were reproducible, causation would be inferred. Confidence regarding causation would be strengthened by double-blind, placebo controlled challenges.

Scientists at Research Triangle Institute have been seeking better methods to assess health effects associated with complex mixtures of chemicals present in indoor air. A number of chemical compounds were selected as representative of a particular newly renovated office building; for example, certain chemicals that were measured outgassing from carpet samples and office partitions. Health effects reported in the TOXNET data base for these individual chemicals were compared with complaints by office workers in the building (Pierson et al. 1990). These are shown in Table 3.2. Health effects reported by the employees were similar to those found in TOXNET, although the literature documents effects at much higher levels of exposure.

The appendix contains an annotated bibliography for health effects that may be related to foods and chemicals. Many, but not all, sources listed were written by clinical ecologists. For certain diseases such as migraine and atopic dermatitis (eczema), traditional practitioners as well are coming to accept that foods may play an important role in certain patients.

This appendix is not intended to be encyclopedic. Rather, it is an attempt to present the range and diversity of diseases for which environmental (food or chemical) origins have been proven or proposed. It is also designed to help the reader identify key articles on particular disorders because many of these articles have appeared in older or less widely circulated journals and would otherwise be difficult to locate.

We have highlighted studies with positive outcomes, that is, those in which a relationship between symptoms and food or chemical exposures was confirmed. Many studies that fail to show an association between symptoms and exposure exclude only a single food from the diet. Those studies of hyperactivity (Kaplan 1989), seizures (Egger et al. 1989), headaches (Egger et al. 1983), and rheumatoid arthritis (Kroker et al.

1984; Marshall et al. 1984) that do show an association tend to use simultaneous avoidance of multiple incitants. Their design should serve as models for future studies in this field.

The majority of the articles discuss foods rather than chemicals as potential factors in disease. Nevertheless, most of the diseases listed here have also been attributed to chemical exposures by some observers. Randolph's observations of patients worked up in an environmental unit are summarized in his books and papers and provide interesting anecdotal accounts of the role chemicals might play in particular conditions.

By presenting this material we are not affirming an environmental cause for these diseases but hoping to alert the reader to that possibility and the need for evaluating such patients in an environmental unit when more traditional approaches have failed. What might seem obvious—that foods and chemicals are not significant factors in most of these disorders—could change if one were to eliminate masking and control for the effects of adaptation.

We cannot overemphasize the importance of avoiding the frequent error of confusing diagnosis and etiology. Terr (1986, 1989a) in his reviews of ecology patients criticizes ecologists for attributing illness in these patients to environmental factors where they clearly had other well-defined clinical diseases such as depression. In a critique of Terr's most recent review of ecology patients, William Meggs (1989b) of East Carolina School of Medicine asserts:

> First, both Dr. Terr and the clinical ecologists consistently confuse diagnosis and etiology. Environmental illness, ecological illness, or similar terms should not be used as a diagnosis, which is the error of the clinical ecologists. Dr. Terr's error is to state that since a patient has another diagnosis, the diagnosis of environmental illness is wrong, and therefore there is no environmental cause of the illness. . . . In his methods section Dr. Terr does not discuss how he determined that the patients' symptoms were not triggered by environmental exposures. Many of the symptoms he lists in Table 4 of his article such as asthma, rhinitis, and dermatitis are known to have an environmental etiology in some patients, and generally accepted methods are available for verification. . . . Correctly diagnosing an autoimmune condition in a patient claiming environmental illness, rather than disproving an environmental etiology, should alert the physician to look for an environmental cause. The claim that psychiatric disorders can be triggered by chemical exposures is worthy of serious scientific study, particularly with increasing rates of depression. . . . Cases of depression related to exposure to furnace fumes were described by Randolph thirty years ago.

The study regarding furnace emissions as a cause of depression is by Randolph (1955).

Table 3-2. Summary of Reported Effects of Indoor Air Pollutants[a]

Body System Effect	AcA	ACE	CUM	DCB	EtB	FOR	STY	TOL	XYL
Eyes									
Irritation[c]	×	×		×	×	×	×	×	×
Irrit. mucous membranes	×					×	×	×	
Conjunctivitis	×	×					×		×
Lacrimation	×	×			×	×			
Diplopia (double vision)[c]		×							
Photophobia	×								
Nose									
Irritation[c]	×	×		×	×	×	×		×
Irrit. mucous membrane						×	×	×	
Runny nose[c]				×					
Respiratory									
Irritation		×			×	×	×	×	×
Pharyngitis		×						×	
Throat irritation[c]				×		×	×		×
Bronchitis	×	×				×			×
Coughing[c]	×					×			
Shortness of breath						×			
Asthmatic reaction						×			
Pulmonary edema	×					×			
Central Nervous									
Tinnitus				×				×	
Headache				×			×	×	
Dizziness[c]		×	×					×	
Depression[c]							×		
Fatigue[c]							×	×	
Confusion[c]							×	×	×

Symptom	AcA	ACE	CUM	DCB	EtB	FOR	STY	TOL	XYL
Drowsiness	×		×						
Vertigo		×	×	×			×		
Slowed reaction time		×							×
Intoxication: Euphoria,			×					×	×
exhileration,		×							
boastfulness, talkative		×							
Incoordination (ataxia)		×	×				×		×
Anasthesia[c]							×	×	
Edema							×		
Weakness		×		×			×		
Skin									
Erythema, irritation			×		×				
Dermatitis	×					×	×		
Blood									
Leukopenia					×			×	
Leukocyctosis					×			×	
Macrocytosis								×	
Reduced erythrocytes								×	
Liver injury				×				×	
Miscellaneous									
Gastritis		×							
Nausea and vomiting		×							
Dysphagia						×			
Menstrual disorders[c]								×	×
Weight loss				×					

[a] Absence of symptoms does not inherently mean that these do not exist for a given compound—only that they were not reported.

[b] Key: AcA = acetaldehyde; ACE = acetone; CUM = cumene (isopropylbenzene); DCB = dichlorobenzene; EtB = ethylbenzene; FOR = formaldehyde; STY = styrene; TOL = toluene; XYL = xylene.

[c] Effects reported associated with the example complex mixture.

Source: Pierson et al. 1990.

Allergists accuse ecologists of overzealously diagnosing environmental illness and overlooking other important medical conditions (Bardana and Montanaro 1989; Terr 1986, 1989a); however, some allergists may have wrongly assumed that a patient's condition that has an accepted medical label cannot have an environmental etiology. Physicians need to be aware of the wide variety of medical conditions for which environmental (either food or chemical) etiologies are being considered. We have attempted to pull together some of the most pertinent articles for the appendix.

If foods and chemicals are responsible for even a modest percentage of the diseases listed in the appendix, the implications are staggering. The trend toward recognition of chemical and food factors in many diseases is growing. Caution must be exercised, however. Perhaps only a subset of patients with a particular illness (for example, rheumatoid arthritis) responds to environmental manipulation. Even one individual who responds positively while fasting in an environmental unit can be an important finding if that finding is reproducible. Thus responses may occur only in a subgroup of sensitive patients. Unless objective testing is limited to that sensitive subgroup, positive results in a few may be diluted by nonresponders, and prevalence studies will not be statistically significant. Clearly, studies of these patients must be carefully constructed if health effects are to be discerned.

How the disorders that have just been discussed relate to the concept of adaptation is unclear at present. Bell and King (1982a) propose that "the chronic symptoms which ecology patients reportedly have with repeated exposures to offending agents may reflect the more insidious, non-adapting changes induced by offending foods and chemicals." For example, individuals may adapt to the *acute* effects of ozone on their upper and lower respiratory tracts, but red blood cell fragility may persist. Others may adapt to the stimulatory effects of caffeine, only to develop fibrocystic disease (Russell 1989; Hindi-Alexander et al. 1985; Boyle et al. 1984) or urticaria (Pola et al. 1988).

Randolph depicts the development of chronic illnesses as in Table 3-3. In the left column are intermittent (acute) responses, and on the right are chronic responses. At the top are stimulatory levels, as discussed in Chapter 2. With continued or repetitive exposures to an incitant, the course of the reactions moves from left to right. Over time, if no intervention occurs, advanced sustained stimulatory responses (upper right) ultimately move toward sustained withdrawal responses (lower right) (Randolph 1987, pp. 248–249). Rea (1988c) speculates that adaptation may indirectly contribute to total body load by covering up (masking) acute reactions with chronic exposure responses so that affected individuals are unaware of the relationship between exposures and the ill-

TABLE 3-3. Environmental-Personal Interrelationships

Intermittent Responses	Levels	Sustained Responses
Mania[a] (agitation, excitement, blackouts, with or without convulsions)	+ + + +	Drug addiction (both natural and synthetic)
Hypomania[a] (hyperresponsiveness, anxiety, panic reactions, mental lapses)	+ + +	Alcoholism (addictive, drinking)
Hyperactivity[a] (restless legs, insomnia, aggressive forceful behavior)	+ +	Obesity (addictive eating)
Stimulation[a] (active, self centered with suppressed symptoms)	+	Absent complaints (the desired way to feel)
Behavior on an even keel, as in homeostasis	0	Behavior on an even keel
Localized physical ecologic manifestations[b] (rhinitis, bronchitis, asthma, dermatitis, gastrointestinal, genitourinary syndromes)	–	Impaired senses of taste and smell, Meniere's syndrome
Systemic physical ecologic manifestations[b] (fatigue, headache, myalgia, arthralgia, arthritis, edema, tachycardia, arrythmia)	– –	Small vessel vasculitis, hypertension, collagen diseases
Brain fag—moderately advanced cerebral syndromes[b] (mood changes, irritability, impaired thinking, reading ability and memory)	– – –	Mental confusion and obfuscation, morose inebriation
Depression—advanced cerebral and behavioral syndromes[b] (confabulation, hallucinosis, obsessions, delusions and temporary amnesia)	– – – –	Dementia, stupor, coma, catatonia, residual amnesia

[a] Specifically adapted stimulatory levels.

[b] Specifically maladapted withdrawal levels.

Source: Randolph, T. and Moss, R., *An Alternative Approach to Allergies,* copyright J. B. Lippincott Co., Philadelphia, PA (1989).

nesses. Smokers, for example, may learn to tolerate the irritating properties of tobacco smoke, but their adaptation only allows them to continue the habit more comfortably, oblivious to the fact that continued exposure may lead to emphysema, cancer, and cardiovascular disease. Patients with multiple chemical sensitivities, on the other hand, frequently experience intense discomfort whenever smoke is present, even in low concentrations. Interestingly, many smokers who quit (deadapt to tobacco) also report acute symptoms with minimal exposure, not unlike those reported by chemically sensitive individuals. This underscores an important point: it is impossible to know how sensitive individuals are to an environmental agent until they are deadapted. Those who appear least sensitive, (smokers, for instance) may in fact be most sensitive with their addiction only masking that sensitivity.

Thus adaptation could play a central role in the development of many medical disorders. Perhaps the best evidence thus far for the existence of adaptation in humans comes from clinical observations of withdrawal symptoms when individuals are removed from their usual exposures and subsequent resolution of formerly chronic symptoms. According to some physicians, this process is viewed optimally in the setting of an environmental unit while patients fast.

In the next chapter we discuss some of the mechanisms that have been proposed for multiple chemical sensitivities.

PART · II

Mechanisms, Diagnosis, and Treatment

CHAPTER 4

Mechanisms of Multiple Chemical Sensitivities

Possible Physiological Mechanisms

A useful review of this topic can be found in Bell (1987b). The limited data available at this time suggest that any mechanism or model that would purport to explain the syndrome of multiple chemical sensitivities would need to address the features most closely associated with this illness:

1. Symptoms involving virtually any system in the body or several systems simultaneously

2. Differing symptoms and severity in different individuals, even those with the same exposure

3. Induction (that is, sensitization) by a wide range of environmental agents

4. Subsequent triggering by lower levels of exposure than those involved in initial induction of the illness

5. Concomitant food intolerances, estimated to occur in a sizable percentage of those with chemical sensitivities

6. "Spreading" of sensitivity to other, often chemically dissimilar substances; each substance may trigger a different constellation of symptoms

7. Adaptation (masking), that is, acclimatization to environmental incitants, both chemical and food, with continued exposure; loss of this tolerance with removal from the incitant(s); and augmented response with reexposure after an appropriate interval (for example, 4 to 7 days)

8. An apparent threshold effect referred to by some (including certain traditional allergists we interviewed) as the patient's *total load*. Total load is a theoretical construct that has been invoked by clinical ecologists to help explain why an individual develops this syndrome at a particular time. Illness is said to occur when the total load of biological, chemical, physical, and psychological stressors exceeds some threshold for the patient. This concept has emerged from clinical observations; no direct experiments have been done to test its validity in humans; however, animal models do exist. The concept aligns with Selye's (1946) work on the general adaptation syndrome.

Randolph knew Selye and was intrigued by his ideas but failed to see their clinical utility. Hans Selye (1977) was concerned with the general response of an organism to stressors. He observed that animals treated with a variety of toxic substances (indeed, Selye's supervisor accused him of spending his entire life studying the pharmacology of dirt) reacted in the same way: all had a generalized response involving increased endocrine activity and adrenal size, reduction of lymphatic tissue including the thymus (where T lymphocytes undergo maturation), and peptic ulcers in the stomach and duodenum). Selye defined stress as the nonspecific response of the body to any demand. Three phases occur:

1. An alarm reaction accompanied by increased adrenocorticotrophic hormone (ACTH) release

2. Resistance, during which demands upon the organism are met with little increase in ACTH or steroid hormone production; this stage corresponds with Randolph's adapted stage

3. Exhaustion, when animals succumb to stress, having expended their adaptive energy

The most characteristic feature of the stress syndrome, according to Selye, is its nonspecificity. All stresses (typhoid, cold, ecstasy, malnutrition) have their own features and causes, but all require the body to adjust to the demand for adaptation. When organisms succumb to excessive stress, their individual manifestations may differ somewhat, but the result is the same: as with a chain, there is always a weakest link, a point at which things are most likely to break down.

Randolph's concept of specific adaptation parallels Selye's, but differs in one key respect: adaptation in a given individual is specific to the incitant. Selye recognized this possibility but chose to focus on the more global aspects of adaptation. In Randolph's view, the accumulation of multiple stressors could overwhelm the organism's ability to adapt. In the exhaustion phase, Selye's general adaptation syndrome and Randolph's concept of specific adaptation coincide. From these ideas emerged the ecologists' concept of total load of stressors or incitants as the determinant of an individual's ability to adapt or failure to adapt. Ecologists consider Randolph's substance-specific and individual-specific view of adaptation to be the clinical counterpart of Selye's general adaptation syndrome (Randolph 1962, pp. 6–8; 1976a).

Rea probably has performed more clinical laboratory tests on chemically sensitive patients than any other clinical ecologist. When we asked him what mechanism he thought was responsible for these patients' illness, he responded, "Which one?" In his view, many interacting factors may be present. No single biochemical or immunological abnormality appears consistently in every patient. Some may have abnormal levels of immunoglobulins, complement, immune complexes, T-cells, B-cells, prostaglandins, kinins, serotonin, histamine, acetylcholine, vitamins, minerals, or detoxification enzymes (such as glutathione peroxidase) (Johnson and Rea 1989). Rea sees a great diversity of patients because he receives referrals of more difficult cases from other physicians. More clearly defined, homogeneous patient groups, such as those from a specific workplace, contaminated community, or tight building, might very well exhibit less variation in their laboratory profiles. (See discussion in Chapter 6.)

Before we examine some of the specific theories that have been proposed to explain multiple chemical sensitivity, three important points must be recognized:

1. The human body is an integrated system that traditionally has been separated into its component parts or systems to facilitate study. Interactions of these parts are necessarily more complex. For example, multiple chemical sensitivities conceivably could involve the entire neuroimmunoendocrine axis. Teasing out the subtle biochemical interactions involved in adaptation to the plethora of substances in the environment may be extremely difficult.

2. Traditional allergists who have studied sensitivity to industrial chemicals have been as baffled as the ecologists in trying to discern a mechanism for hyperreactivity. Butcher and co-workers (1982) remarked upon the continuing controversy over the mechanism for isocyanate hyperreactivity. Although an immunological theory has

been proposed, specific antibody is demonstrable in only 15 to 20 percent of reactive individuals. That antibodies also may persist beyond loss of reactivity casts doubt upon their role. More recently, Stankus, Salvaggio and associates (1988) demonstrated airway hyperreactivity to cigarette smoke among asthmatics who lacked specific IgE to tobacco smoke components. They report that the mechanism(s) behind this hyperreactivity remain unclear. These observations concerning the effects of cigarette smoke on some individuals parallel similar observations by clinical ecologists.

3. Although knowledge of the mechanism of a disease may be useful for developing better therapies, such knowledge is not a prerequisite for intervention. Preventing the development of multiple chemical sensitivities in those not yet afflicted may be possible by controlling environmental exposures that cause the initial sensitization.

The most frequently cited theories to explain chemical sensitivity involve the nervous system, the immune system, or the interaction between them because these two systems most clearly link the external environment and the internal milieu (Bell 1982). The rapid responsiveness of these systems also makes them attractive candidates because symptoms of food or chemical sensitivity have been reported to develop within seconds of exposure. As early as the 1940s and 1950s, the allergist Coca recommended sympathectomies (surgical interruption of certain sympathetic nerve pathways) in some cases of multiple food sensitivities, but benefits were often short-lived (Randolph 1987).

David Ozonoff (1989), professor of medicine and chief, Environmental Health Section, Boston University School of Public Health, suggests that because low levels of exposure do not trigger symptoms in everyone, perhaps a small initiating stimulus occurs, which the body of the chemically sensitive patient then amplifies or magnifies. In the case of multiple chemical sensitivities, the nervous system, the immune system, or both might amplify an external signal. Many chemicals, such as polybrominated biphenyls (PBBs) and trichloroethylene, affect both the nervous system and the immune system. Until 1980, the idea of a possible direct communication between the nervous and immune systems was widely debated. Subsequently, the existence of a neuroimmunoendocrine axis has been increasingly realized. Payan (1989, Payan et al. 1986) cites several discoveries that have helped to confirm the presence of two-way communication between the nervous and immune systems.

1. Studies show that neuropeptides (for example, substance P and somatostatin) and the nerve ganglia from which they arise project into immunological tissues.

2. Receptors for these neuropeptides occur on immunologically active leukocytes.

3. Certain immunologically active substances such as the interleukins can activate or be activated by cells in the nervous system.

4. Electrolytic lesions in the hypothalamus of animals produce distinct alterations in antibody production as well as abnormalities in the number and role of natural killer cells and T-lymphocytes. These alterations occur because of the interruption of a network of noradrenergic and peptidergic fibers that project into lymphoid tissues, including the thymus, spleen, Peyer's patches of the intestine, and bone marrow.

Therefore, the endocrine, immune, and nervous systems, once perceived as separate compartments, are increasingly recognized as interconnected.

Mechanisms Involving the Limbic System

The hypothalamus (part of the limbic system) has attracted considerable attention because it is the focal point in the brain where the immune, nervous, and endocrine systems interact (Bell 1982). Bell notes that assuming a direct cause-and-effect relationship would be premature, but that the hypothalamus could mediate food and chemical addictions in patients with multiple chemical sensitivities. The olfactory system has known links to the hypothalamus and other parts of the limbic system, which has led Bell (1982) to speculate that "the olfactory system, hypothalamus and limbic system pathways would provide the neural circuitry by which adverse food and chemical reactions could trigger certain neural, psychological and psychiatric abnormalities." Many different chemicals have been reported by clinical ecologists to trigger food cravings, binges, violence, or hypersexual activity. A model involving the hypothalamus could help to explain such behavioral changes in response to chemical exposures.

Some authors have alleged that psychological conditioning to odors is responsible for patients' reactions to chemicals. Of course, odor conditioning may occur in selected cases. (See the next section for a discussion of psychogenic mechanisms.) However, physiological mechanisms involving the limbic system may be at work. A direct pathway from the oropharynx to the brain and hypothalamic and limbic region has been demonstrated in rats (Kare 1968; Maller et al. 1967). Substances placed in the oropharynx migrated to the brain in minutes via a pathway other than the blood stream and in higher concentrations than if administered via the gastrointestinal tract, suggesting a direct route from mouth (or nose) to brain. Similarly, Shipley (1985) showed that inhaled substances that contact the nasal epithelium may cross into the brain and be distributed widely via transneuronal (through the nerve cell) transport. Thus, molecules that are inhaled and contact the olfactory apparatus could influence functions in other parts of the brain.

Bell (1990), a psychiatrist, notes that individuals who are shy tend to be more atopic (have a greater tendency to manifest allergies). She hypothesizes that chemical mediators, for example, histamine, VIP (vasoactive intestinal peptide), and prostaglandins, released in the nose in response to environmental agents may undergo transneuronal transport to the limbic system, temporal lobe, and other parts of the brain and there influence thought, mood, and personality traits such as shyness.

Ryan and co-workers (1988) studied 17 workers who attributed changes in thought processes, particularly memory and concentration difficulties, or changes in mood to their exposure to solvents. Those workers with "cacosmia" (a heightened sensitivity to odors) performed most poorly on neurobehavioral tests requiring verbal learning or visual memory. Although olfactory functioning was not tested objectively in this study, the authors felt their findings supported a hypothesis that chronic solvent exposure may affect the "rhinencephalic structures" (the primitive "smell" brain), the evolutionary precursor of the limbic system.

This phylogenetically ancient part of the brain (Fig. 4-1) is present in all mammals. It influences the organism's interaction with its environment in many subtle ways essential for preservation of the individual, its offspring, and the species. *Limbus* (Latin for "margin" or "rim") refers to its appearing like a rim around the edge of the cerebral hemispheres. Figure 4-2 shows its component parts. Note the close anatomical relationship to the olfactory bulb. Strong odors and even milder ones may provoke increased electrical activity in the amygdala and hippocampal areas of the limbic system (Monroe 1986). Subsensory exposure to chemicals can cause protracted, if not permanent, alterations in the electrical activity of the brain, beginning first with the most sensitive structures, particularly that portion of the amygdala that analyzes odors (Bokina 1976).

The amygdala is involved in feelings and activities related to self-preservation, such as searching for food, feeding, fighting, and self-protection (MacLean 1986). The cingulate gyrus appears to influence maternal care and nursing, separation cries between mother and offspring, and playful behavior, including wit and humor (MacLean 1986). The septum involves feeling and expression relating to procreation. Lesions in the septal area may cause hyperresponsiveness to physical stimuli (such as touching, sounds, or temperature changes), hyperemotionality, loss of motivation, excessive sugar and water intake, and fear of unfamiliar situations (Isaacson 1982).

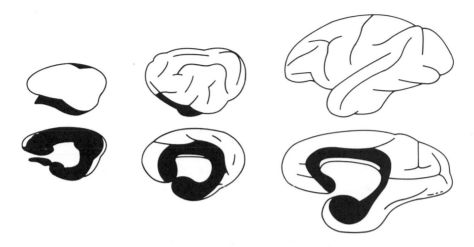

FIGURE 4-1. *The cortex of the paleomammalian brain (limbic system) is contained in the great limbic lobe surrounding the brain stem. Shown in black is the location and relative size of the limbic lobe in the brains of the rabbit, cat, and monkey; the ring of limbic cortex is found as a common denominator in the brains of all mammals. The surrounding cortex of the neomammalian brain which undergoes a rapid expansion in evolution is shown in white.*
Source: *MacLean, P. D., "The Brain in Relation to Empathy and Medical Education,"* Journal of Nervous and Mental Disease *(1967) 144(5):374–382: Williams & Wilkins, Baltimore, Maryland, p. 377.*

The hippocampus appears important for laying down new memories and thus is essential for learning (Gilman 1982). Hippocampal lesions may cause difficulty in retaining recent memories (Isaacson 1982). The hippocampus, at the intersection of numerous neural pathways and in a critical position to affect the transfer of information from one brain region to another, acts as an information switching center. Learning and memory decrements are a frequent consequence of exposure to toxic substances, and some researchers view the hippocampus as a prime target for such toxins (NAS 1990, Walsh 1988). Damage to the hippocampus itself, or to nerves leading to or from it, may adversely affect the synthesis, storage, release, or inactivation of the excitatory and inhibitory amino acids that serve as neurotransmitters in this region of the brain. Toxins may disrupt the delicate balance of these amino acids, perhaps leading to the release of a flood of excitatory neurotransmitters that damage neighboring cells, a phenomenon that has been called *excitotoxicity* (U.S. Congress 1990). Relatively small perturbations of hippocampal function may have large and long-lasting effects upon behavior and cognition (Walsh 1988).

The most vital component of the limbic system, the hypothalamus,

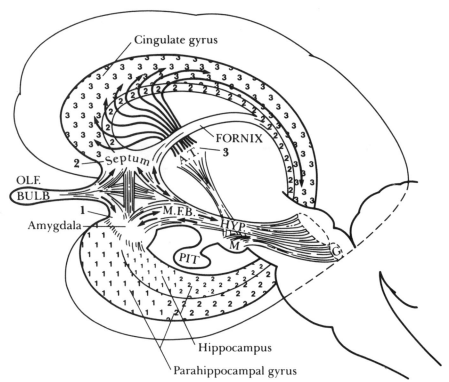

FIGURE 4-2.   *Three major subdivisions of the limbic system. The small numerals 1, 2, and 3 overlie, respectively, the amygdaloid, septal, and thalamocingulate divisions. The corresponding large numerals identify connecting nuclei in the amygdala, septum, and anterior thalamus. Abbreviations: AT, anterior thalamic nuclei; G, tegmental nuclei of Gudden; HYP, hypothalamus; M, mammillary bodies; MFB, median forebrain bundle; PIT, pituitary; OLF, olfactory.*
Source: MacLean, P. D., "A Triune Concept of the Brain and Behavior," in Boag, T., and Campbell, D., The Hincks Memorial Lectures (1973), University of Toronto Press, Toronto, Ontario, p. 15.

governs: (1) body temperature via vasoconstriction, shivering, vasodilation, sweating, fever, and behaviors such as moving to a cooler or warmer environment or putting on or taking off clothing; (2) reproductive physiology and behavior; (3) feeding, drinking, digestive, and metabolic activities, including water balance, addictive eating leading to obesity, and complete refusal of food and water leading to death; (4) aggressive behavior, including such physical manifestations of emotion as increased heart rate, elevated blood pressure, dry mouth, and gastrointestinal responses (Gilman 1982).

The hypothalamus is also the locus at which sympathetic and parasympathetic nervous systems converge. Many symptoms experienced by patients with food and chemical sensitivities relate to the autonomic (sympathetic and parasympathetic) nervous systems; for example, altered smooth muscle tone produces Raynaud's phenomenon, diarrhea, constipation, and other symptoms. Recently, Rea and his co-workers acquired an iriscorder (to be distinguished from iridology) from the Japanese who have used this instrument to measure pupillary reactivity in persons with organophosphate pesticide toxicity. A brief pulse of intense light evokes pupillary constriction (a parasympathetic response) followed by dilation (a sympathetic response). With the aid of this device, they are attempting to monitor objectively sympathetic and parasympathetic nerve function in persons with chemical sensitivities.

The hypothalamus appears to influence anaphylaxis and other aspects of immunity (Stein 1981). Likewise, antigens may affect electrical activity in the hypothalamus (Besedovsky 1977).

Thoughts arising in the cerebral cortex that have strong emotional overtones can trigger hypothalamic responses and recreate the physical effects associated with intense anger, fear, and other feelings. To implement its effects, the hypothalamus not only has a direct electrical output to the nervous system but also produces its own hormones, many of which stimulate or inhibit the pituitary's production of hormones (Gilman 1982).

Corwin (1978) describes the complexity and delicacy of hypothalamic function.

> Imagine, if you will, a chemical laboratory set up to monitor a stream of fluid continuously. This laboratory is equipped to perform analyses for simple substances such as acids, bases, and salts, ions, such as sodium, potassium, calcium, and chloride, and more complex substances such as glucose and cholesterol, simple hormones such as adrenaline and thyroxine, more complex hormones such as the peptide hormones. This laboratory has a built-in computer which evaluates the balance between all these substances and controls this balance so that in case one is formed in excess, the valves can be tightened electrically to decrease the production or to generate an antagonist. In addition, this laboratory has the means for the synthesis of organic chemicals which can be released into the flowing stream of fluid at appropriate points to alter the action of the way stations producing the desired or undesired materials. . . . The human body has its analytical laboratory, computer controller, and hormone factory compressed into a few grams of hypothalamus, a true marvel of microminiaturization.

Most of the neural input to the hypothalamus comes from the nearby limbic and olfactory areas (Isaacson 1982). Lesions in the limbic region may be associated with irrational fears, feelings of strangeness or unreality, wishing to be alone, and sadness (MacLean 1967). A feeling of being out of touch with or out of control of one's feelings and thoughts, not unlike that described by many patients with chemical sensitivity, may be perceived.

Doane (1986) describes potential difficulties for patients with limbic dysfunction.

> Activity controlled by the limbic system may seem largely irrational and often is not perceived within one's self in ways that are easily understood or communicated in verbal language. These observations do not detract, however, from the reality of limbic determinism in human psychic functions and psychiatric disorders.

The dynamic involvement of the hypothalamus and limbic system in virtually every aspect of human physiology and behavior makes injury to these structures an intriguing hypothesis to explain chemical sensitivity's myriad manifestations. Rich neural connections lie between the olfactory system and the limbic and temporal regions of the brain. Surgical or epileptic patients with damage to the limbic or medial temporal portions of the brain may have persistent alterations in odor perception (for example, an unusual smell that characteristically precedes seizure activity) as well as learning and memory difficulties (Ryan 1988).

Bell (1990) hypothesizes that chemically sensitive patients may have olfactory-limbic-temporal pathways that are more easily "kindled." In other words, a small signal or insult would more readily trigger firing of nerve cells in brain regions where kindling was present. Kindling might be enhanced by genetic endowment, prior environmental exposures, psychological stress, hormonal variations, or other factors. Unlike surgical ablation, which destroys a brain area, kindling is a kind of stimulatory lesion (Girgis 1986). Stimulation of the amygdala with electrodes may elicit rage or loss of control of emotions, a phenomenon frequently reported by patients with multiple chemical sensitivities.

Kindling has been described previously in the context of seizures. The amygdala, for example, which is particularly susceptible to electrical discharge following either electrical (Girgis 1986) or chemical provocation (Bokina 1976), is subject to long-lasting alteration when given repeated stimuli. Very potent or repeated stimuli, whether electrical or chemical, may permanently augment the tendency for neurons to fire in the presence of future stimuli, even when challenged with much lower levels than those originally involved. Girgis (1986) reports a decrease in acetylcholinesterase (AChE), an enzyme that breaks down the neurotransmitter acetylcholine in junctions between nerve cells, that parallels the increase in supersensitivity to stimuli. The limbic system is especially rich in AChE, which is strongly bound to the nerve cell membranes and very stable. The AChE may play a protective role by enzymatically maintaining acetylcholine concentrations at nerve junctions within safe bounds and protecting susceptible cells in the limbic system from developing "bizarre sensitivity" (Girgis 1986). Interestingly, physicians who treat patients with multiple chemical sensitivities have noted some of the most severe and debilitating exposures for these patients have been to organophosphate pesticides, which inhibit AChE.

Bokina (1976) found impaired speed of execution and coordination of complex motor processes in humans repeatedly exposed to carbon disulfide for 10- to 15-minute intervals at subsensory levels. Animals primed by high concentrations of various chemicals (such as formaldehyde and ozone) and subsequently reexposed to low concentrations of the same chemicals showed an increased tendency toward paroxysmal electrical discharge in the amygdala (Bokina 1976). Bokina observed that although the chemicals he used to sensitize the animals were *different in terms of their structure and physical and chemical properties, their effects upon the limbic system were remarkably similar.*

Kindling could help to explain the apparent loss of adaptive capacity in multiple chemical sensitivity. Formerly well-tolerated low-level exposures to, for example, tobacco smoke or perfume might trigger symptoms in individuals whose limbic areas have been kindled by a prior exposure. Likewise, spreading of sensitivities to chemically unrelated substances might be understood on this basis.

One intriguing aspect of the limbic system as a mechanism for multiple chemical sensitivities is its responsiveness to both chemical and cortical stimuli. Therefore, conscious thought processes and emotional states influence limbic activity just as chemical or physical stimuli can. The former may be under more or less conscious control of the individual, whereas the latter are almost entirely unconscious and automatic. However, conscious efforts that play into the delicate circuitry of the limbic system may be able to alter or suppress concurrent electrical activity evoked by environmental agents. Nevertheless, very potent exposures may not be susceptible to conscious will. Some patients with chemical sensitivities report being able to "will" their way out of a mild reaction to a food or chemical and attempt to control their symptoms in this manner. Most say such efforts do not work for their most problematic incitants. In fact, the ability to exercise any conscious effort, even that of simply getting away from the exposure or taking alkali salts or a neutralizing dose, may be lost during a reaction. Monroe (1986) reported the case of a man for whom exposure to the odor of stale beer caused greatly increased electrical activity in the limbic system (amygdala and hippocampal areas). Various memories, some associated with beer, also increased electrical activity in the same region. However, simple arithmetic computations would immediately stop such activity. There-fore, conscious thought processes could override preexisting activity in the limbic system.

An intriguing example of the competing effects of exposure and psy-chological state has been reported by Sanderson (1989; for more detail see in the appendix "Neurobehavioral and Psychiatric Manifestations"). Carbon dioxide at levels greater than 5 percent in the air has been shown to induce panic attacks ("fight or flight" responses depend upon limbic activity) in patients suffering from panic disorder. While this effect is not chemical sensitivity, the fact that patients in this study who believed that they had control over the carbon dioxide level to which they were exposed had fewer and less intense panic disorder symptoms suggests that psychological factors (the illusion of control) can indeed mitigate the biological response to an environmental stressor.

Thus, experimental evidence suggests a delicate interplay occurring in the limbic region. Conceivably, chemicals contacting olfactory nerve projections in the nose could either be transported into or relay electrical signals to the limbic region, leading to a vast array of symptoms. Like-wise, thought processes and mood states trigger limbic activity or may, in some cases, interrupt preexisting limbic activity. At present, however, no evidence suggests that limbic activity triggered by environmental exposures can be entirely overcome by psychological interventions.

Immunologic Mechanisms

Immunological alterations are another possible explanation for multiple chemical sensitivities. Most of us have been taught that the immune system evolved to defend our bodies against microorganisms and other "foreign invaders." In truth, the immune system may have evolved to help control the body's internal milieu. Thus, its purpose is not simply to ward off infections but also to carry out precise regulatory interactions between the immune system, endocrine system, and nervous system.

Scientists are only beginning to learn which chemicals affect our im-mune system and what those effects mean in terms of our health. Ani-mal experiments demonstrate immunotoxicity from halogenated aromatics, heavy metals, and organochlorine pesticides (Cone et al. 1987). Accidental human exposures to aldicarb, polybrominated bi-phenyls (PBBs), dioxin, and other toxins also provide data that chemi-cals can impact the immune system. Volumes, for example, Sharma (1981), have been written on the subject of immunotoxicology. Descotes (1986) has attempted to catalog the extensive published literature on the immunomodulatory action of chemicals and drugs. Of special con-cern to allergists and some clinical ecologists have been Levin and

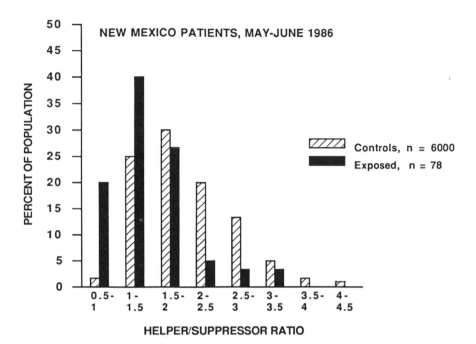

FIGURE 4-3. *New Mexico patients, May–June 1986. Helper/suppressor ratios obtained by standard clinical laboratory procedures in 78 injured workers from a computer chip manufacturing plant in Albuquerque, New Mexico, compared with the standard laboratory control population of 6,000 randomly selected asymptomatic people. The exposed population is statistically significantly different from the controls (chi-square = 39.34063: p = 2.62 × 10< − 6>).* Reprinted with permission from Levin, A. and V. Byers, "Environmental Illness: A Disorder of Immune Regulation," in Workers with Multiple Chemical Sensitivities, M. Cullen, Ed. *(copyright 1987, Hanley & Belfus, Inc., Philadelphia, PA), p. 672.*

Byers's (1987) assertions that environmental illness is a disorder of immune regulation. These authors point to decreased T-lymphocyte helper-suppressor ratios in four different populations exposed to environmental toxins. Figures 4-3 through 4-6 depict helper-suppressor ratios for these four groups.

Note that all four figures show a shift to the left (decrease) of the ratio of helper to suppressor T-lymphocytes.

The Woburn, Massachusetts, data (Fig. 4-5) is taken from 25 surviving family members of leukemia patients, all of whom drank water from wells contaminated with industrial solvents. Not only did these individuals have a statistically significant reduction in their T-cell helper-to-suppressor ratios (1.49 versus 1.94 in age- and sex-matched asymptomatic controls, p <0.01) but also 48 percent (11 of 23) tested positive for autoantibodies. In addition, 88 percent (22) had frequent or chronic sinusitis or rhinitis, and 52 percent (13) had gastrointestinal complaints

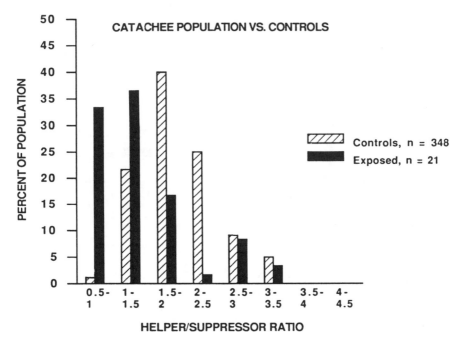

FIGURE 4-4. Catachee population vs. controls. Helper/suppressor ratios obtained by standard clinical laboratory procedures on 21 environmentally ill patients who were domestically exposed to high levels of polychlorinated biphenyls (PCBs) over a period of 5 to 10 years in Catachee, South Carolina, compared with the standard laboratory control population of 348 asymptomatic individuals. The exposed population is statistically significantly different from the controls (chi-square = 63.48208: p = 1.37 × 10<—6>). Reprinted with permission from Levin, A. and V. Byers, *"Environmental Illness: A Disorder of Immune Regulation,"* in Workers with Multiple Chemical Sensitivities, *M. Cullen, Ed. (copyright 1987, Hanley & Belfus, Inc., Philadelphia, PA), p. 673.*

often described as irritable bowel syndrome. Rashes were frequent. Fourteen adults complained of rapid heart rate at rest, palpitation, or near syncope; of 11 who underwent cardiac workups, eight had multi-focal premature ventricular contractions, and six were felt to need cardiac medications (Byers et al. 1988).

What is remarkable are the many similarities between the Woburn data and data gathered by Johnson and Rea (1989) on patients who have been worked up in the ecologists' environmental unit in Dallas. Of 150 ecology patients, 19 percent were positive for antinuclear antibodies. Many others had antithyroglobulin or other autoantibodies. In addition, the polysymptomatic complaints of the Woburn study group resemble those of the ecology patients. However, differences are present too. In 70 ecology patients with vascular dysfunction, the T_4-T_8 (helper-suppressor) ratio was *increased* (2.20) versus 60 controls (1.70) ($p = 0.001$).

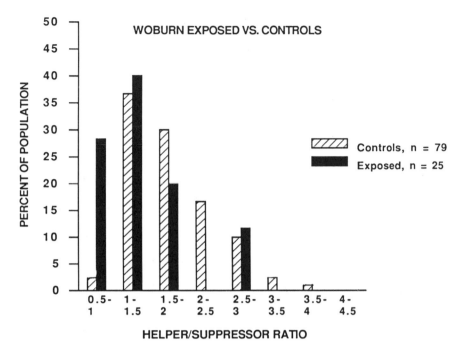

FIGURE 4-5.   Woburn exposed population vs. controls. Helper/suppressor ratios obtained by standard clinical laboratory procedures on 25 environmentally ill patients from Woburn, Massachusetts, who were domestically exposed to trichloroethylene (TCE) over a period of 5 to 10 years compared with age and sex matched asymptomatic controls. The exposed population was statistically significantly different from the controls (chi-square = 42.18912: p = <1 × 10 <—8>). This control population is not significantly different from the standard laboratory controls used in the other studies. Reprinted with permission from Levin, A. and V. Byers, "Environmental Illness: A Disorder of Immune Regulation," in Workers with Multiple Chemical Sensitivities, *M. Cullen, Ed. (copyright 1987, Hanley & Belfus, Inc., Philadelphia, PA), p. 674.*

Seven rheumatoid arthritis patients showed similar increases in T_4-T_8, whereas 27 asthmatics showed no significant differences from controls. Why certain individuals have increased T_4-T_8 ratios while others have decreased ratios is unclear. Perhaps differences exist in the kinds of patients in these studies, the exact nature of their exposures, or the time elapsed since exposure. Interestingly, cigarette smoking, which is well recognized for its long-term adverse health consequences, recently has been linked to an increased number of T_4 (helper) cells (p = 0.002) and an increased T_4-T_8 ratio (p = 0.02) (Tollerud et al. 1989).

Such data warrant further studies employing carefully matched controls. Levin's work has stirred considerable controversy among allergists and clinical ecologists. His focus on the immune system has drawn allergists and immunologists into the fray because it is their area of

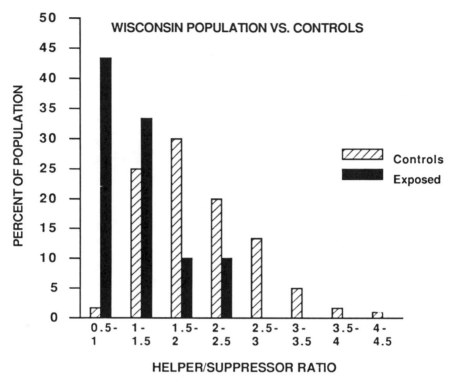

FIGURE 4-6.   *Wisconsin population vs. controls. Helper/suppressor ratios obtained by standard clinical laboratory procedures on 10 environmentally ill patients from rural Wisconsin who were domestically exposed to a variety of industrial dyes, solvents, and pesticides over a 5 to 10 year period compared to the standard laboratory control of 6,000 randomly selected asymptomatic people. The exposed are significantly different from the controls (chi-square = 73.58482:* p = 4.77 × 10 <— 6>). Reprinted with permission from Levin, A. and V. Byers, "Environmental Illness: A Disorder of Immune Regulation,"* in Workers with Multiple Chemical Sensitivities, M. Cullen, Ed. *(copyright 1987, Hanley & Belfus, Inc., Philadelphia, PA), p. 675.*

specialization. Levin and traditional allergists often serve as expert witnesses on opposing sides in lawsuits and disability evaluations. Terr (1986) asserts that immune parameters of patients who have seen clinical ecologists fall within expected normal ranges "except for several patients who had immunoglobulin (IgA) and lymphocyte levels above the normal range, reflecting a history of infections." Levin (1989) counters by arguing that only 2.5 percent of the population would be expected to fall outside the normal range, whereas in Terr's data 20 to 30 percent of these patients fall outside the normal range.

As can be seen from Figures 4-3 through 4-6, individual data points (a single individual's helper-suppressor ratio) may be difficult to interpret as normal or abnormal because the ranges for normal data are quite wide. However, when one looks at an entire exposed population, the data appear to be skewed to the left, that is, toward a *reduced* helper-suppressor ratio. Levin (1989) suggested about some recent data that the reduced helper-suppressor T-lymphocyte ratios seen in many chemically exposed individuals may be the result of increased numbers of cytotoxic lymphocytes in the suppressor cell population of these patients. Such cytotoxic lymphocytes could be "reactively cloned in response to a somatically transformed cell," that is, a cell somehow transformed by a chemical agent.

Similarly, Broughton and associates (1988) report T-lymphocyte activation, particularly increases in Ta1 positive T-lymphocytes, in persons exposed to formaldehyde, even after exposure has ceased. The Ta1 positive cells are elevated in certain autoimmune disorders including multiple sclerosis (Hafler 1985) and juvenile-onset diabetes (Jackson 1982) and after immunization (Yu 1980). These activated T-lymphocytes may serve as an index of immunological stimulation (Yu 1980). Broughton and co-workers (1988) propose that lymphocyte activation may continue in spite of formaldehyde avoidance by these chemically sensitive individuals as a result of the emergence of cross-sensitivities to other environmental chemicals that are not being avoided.

The idea that relatively low-molecular-weight chemicals can somehow alter native protein, perhaps by acting as haptens, and elicit a sort of autoimmune response to that altered protein is gaining support. Formaldehyde (Thrasher et al. 1987), trimellitic anhydride (Akiyama et al. 1984), isocyanate (Butcher et al. 1982), hydantoins (Kammuller et al. 1988), which are present in many drugs and foods, and hydrazine (Reidenberg et al. 1983), which occurs in mushrooms, plastics, pesticides, tobacco smoke, and various drugs, have all been reputed to cause immune derangement, possibly by such a mechanism.

Broughton, and Thrasher (1988) have studied more than 200 cases involving formaldehyde exposure and reported the development of antibodies to formaldehyde-albumin conjugates, evidence of immune system activation (activation marker Ta1 on T-lymphocytes), low titers of a variety of autoantibodies, and altered IL-1 (interleukin) production in these individuals, suggestive of "subtle but chronic activation of the immune system" (Broughton et al. 1990). They state that similar alterations occur in patients exposed to chlordane (a termiticide) and solvents in drinking water. Testing blood from symptomatic patients with a history of chemical exposure, Broughton and Thrasher noted a much higher incidence of autoantibodies among these patients than among controls (Broughton 1990). Individuals exposed to formaldehyde, trichloroethylene, and chlordane were tested for antinuclear antibody

(ANA) and autoantibodies to parietal cells, smooth muscle, brush border, mitochondria, and myelin. The clinical significance of some of these antibodies, particularly in low titers, is not known, but the differences between exposed and unexposed groups are striking and warrant further investigation (Table 4-1). Exposed groups were three to four times more likely than controls to have one or more autoantibodies present. In addition, the incidence of autoantibodies appeared higher when exposure was ongoing than when some time had elapsed. Many such chemicals are metabolized in the liver via the cytochrome P450 enzyme system and excreted in the urine. However, these authors speculate, highly reactive intermediate compounds, such as epoxides, formed during processing may damage liver cells and signal immune system cells to enter the area and clean up the debris. Macrophages (the "trash collector" cells of the immune system) produce interleukin-1, which can evoke flulike symptoms. Cell fragments, previously hidden to the immune system, may also trigger autoantibody production.

Antibodies to albumin conjugates of formaldehyde, tolulene diisocyanate, and trimellitic anhydride were reported in symptomatic workers in a newly remodeled building (Thrasher et al. 1989). Patterson and co-workers (1989) at Northwestern University Medical School analyzed blood from symptomatic individuals exposed to formaldehyde via inhalation and from hemodialysis patients who had intravenous exposure to formaldehyde. In striking contrast to Broughton and associates, they found no correlation between the presence of IgG antibodies to either formaldehyde or formaldehyde conjugated to albumin and the symptoms from formaldehyde exposure.

Some individuals exposed to toluene diisocyanate (TDI), used in the manufacture of urethane foams and plastics, develop respiratory difficulties and may experience symptoms upon reexposure to even very low concentrations of TDI. Yet, the majority of TDI-sensitive individuals do not have antibodies to TDI in their blood. Conversely, the presence of antibodies to TDI in the blood is felt to reflect prior exposure, not illness resulting from that exposure. Some, however, argue that antibodies to foreign chemicals do not occur naturally and that subclinical effects— effects not detectable using current diagnostic tools but nevertheless real —may be occurring.

Future governmental and scientific investigations must include measurement of T- and B-cell numbers, lymphocyte activation, and other relevant immune parameters as possible indices of toxicity. Levin and others have helped draw attention to the need for these data.

Clinical ecologists have examined other indicators of immune system function for their relevance. Commonly, IgE levels are normal or even low in their patients, but some are elevated. According to ecologists,

TABLE 4-1. Autoantibody Presence Among Chemically Exposed Groups

Chemical	Symptoms Reported	Autoantibodies Present[a]	% of These Groups Reporting Symptoms						
			Controls (n = 28)	Mobile-home Dwellers (n = 19)	Office Workers (n = 20)	Occupationally exposed (n = 6) Workers	Currently Exposed (n = 39)	Removed from Exposure (2 years) (n = 39)	Exposed (n = 20)
Formaldehyde	Mucosal irritation, fatigue, flu-like syndrome	1 or more	21	89	80	66			
		2 or more	7	58	45	33			
		3 or more	0	37	15	33			
		4 or more	0	0	0	0			
Trichloroethylene[b]	Fatigue, flu-like syndrome, cognitive difficulties	1 or more	20				91	41.2	
		2 or more	0				43	26	
		3 or more	0				30	12.8	
		4 or more	0				0	0	
Chlordane[c]	Fatigue, flu-like syndrome, cognitive difficulties	1 or more	21						95
		2 or more	7						60
		3 or more	0						35
		4 or more	0						10

[a] Autoantibodies measured for the formaldehyde and chlordane-exposed control groups were ANA (antinuclear antibody) and antiparietal cell, brush order, mitochondria, and smooth muscle. For the trichloroethylene-exposed and control groups, antimyelin antibodies were also measured.

[b] Exposed through drinking water.

[c] Exposed in individuals' homes.

Sources: Broughton, A., Thrasher, J. D., Personal communication, 1990. Broughton A., Thrasher, J. D., Madison, R., "Chronic Health Effects and Immunological Alterations Associated with Exposure to Pesticides," *Comments Toxicology* (in press), 1990. Thrasher, J. D., Broughton, A., Madison, R., "Immune Activation and Autoantibodies in Humans with Long-term Inhalation Exposure to Formaldehyde," *Archives of Environmental Health* (in press, July/August), 1990.

abnormal activation of the complement system may occur; increased autoantibodies may be present. Lymphokines, prostaglandins, kinins, and a host of other mediators may be affected, but, again, none of these applies for all patients (Johnson and Rea 1989).

McGovern (1983), a clinical ecologist, challenged six normal controls and six patients who had multisystem clinical syndromes with foods or chemicals to which they were sensitive and monitored prechallenge and postchallenge blood levels of serotonin, histamine, epinephrine, norepinephrine, dopamine, immunoglobulins, immune complexes, complement, and prostaglandins. Patients included five females and one male, 25 to 75 years of age. Absolute lymphocyte counts for all patients were low or at the low end of normal ranges, that is, 700 to 1100 (normal range: 900 to 2900). Four patients were tested by feeding them a single food to which they were sensitive; one was exposed to 1 ppm of phenol for 5 minutes, and another was exposed to the emissions of a photocopy machine for 5 minutes. Controls underwent identical challenges but reportedly had no symptoms. Unfortunately, challenges were not blinded. Within 15 to 30 minutes after challenge, all patients developed some abnormal *physical findings,* for example, asthma, tachycardia, ataxia, ophthalmoplegia, finger swelling, cough, rhinitis, or shaking chills. Symptoms persisted for 2 to 8 hours after challenge. The results are shown in Figure 4-7.

From the graphs, levels of serotonin, histamine, complement, and immune complexes following provocative challenge appear to be more stable in controls, varying no more than about 10 percent from baseline, except for an early rise in serotonin in controls. In contrast, patients' responses appear far more variable.

The authors speculate that the patients appeared to be having their reactions via various immunological pathways, some type I (IgE-mediated), others type III (IgG-mediated), and some both. Drawing conclusions regarding mechanisms from this paper is difficult, but certainly future challenge studies, preferably blinded, will need to investigate alterations in a panoply of biochemical and immunological markers. Studies of this kind require an enormous amount of preparation and involve costly laboratory analyses, but they are needed to document reactions and elucidate mechanisms.

An intriguing paper concerning the effects of aldicarb (a widely used carbamate insecticide and nematocide) on the immune system of mice demonstrated that aldicarb in the drinking water suppressed the immune response (to sheep red blood cells) more at 1 ppb than at 1,000 ppb (Olson et al. 1987)! This result is a surprising departure from classical toxicological dose-response curves, where dose and toxicity increase together (see Chapter 1). The experiment was carried out several times with two mouse strains and two sources of aldicarb, with the same result. The animals did not die or develop the opportunistic infections usually associated with immune deficiency; however, the authors comment that "such animals will usually not survive a frank challenge with a virulent microorganism." They speculate on the reason for the inverse dose-response curve for aldicarb:

> This phenomenon may be associated with dose related detoxification/elimination in the intestinal tract or body, differential rates of clearance by the kidneys, or possibly the clearance of antigen aided by antibody (induced through conjugation of the chemical to naturally occurring proteins and followed by elicitation of specific antibodies (Olson et al. 1987).

Conceivably, then, lower levels of toxic substances could be more damaging than higher levels, perhaps because damage from the former is so slight that usual cell repair mechanisms are not triggered and the damage becomes permanent.

Biochemical Mechanisms

Rea and other ecologists have noted vitamin and mineral abnormalities in many of their patients (Johnson and Rea 1989; Rogers 1990). Their detractors argue that these patients are often sick, debilitated, and malnourished, and therefore such findings are not surprising. Such a contention is difficult to disprove, even if it were incorrect.

Individuals who have defective enzyme detoxification systems may be more susceptible to low level exposures. Ecologist Rogers reasons that chemically sensitive individuals must have defective detoxification pathways, because others in the same environment tolerate the same exposures without symptoms. Rea has noted that many of his chemically sensitive patients have decreased levels of detoxifying enzymes, such as glutathione peroxidase. This possibility is particularly intriguing because such enzyme systems are inducible (that is, can be stimulated) and thus might conform to an adaptation hypothesis. Scadding and associates (1988) noted poor sulfoxidation ability in 58 of 74 patients with well-defined reactions to foods versus 67 of 200 normal controls ($p < 0.005$). Similarly, Reidenberg and co-workers (1983) reported the case of a laboratory technician who developed a lupuslike disease in response to hydrazine. She was genetically a slow acetylator, which, they felt, might have predisposed her to developing a lupuslike disorder after sufficient exposure to an inciting chemical. A deficiency of one or more particular enzymes could help to explain why some

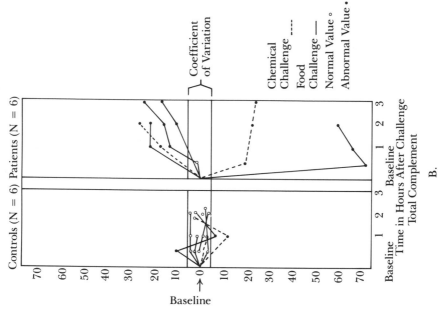

Change From Baseline Levels of CH-100 After Challenge, %

B.

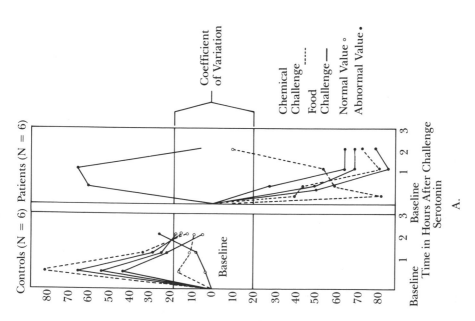

Change From Baseline Level of Serotonin After Challenge, %

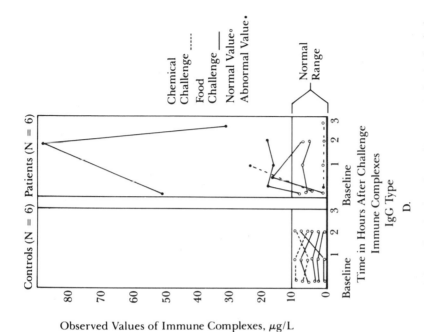

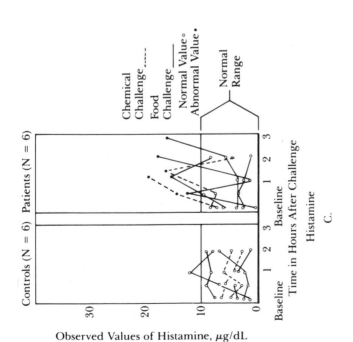

FIGURE 4-7. *Effects of food and chemical challenges on blood-based indicators. A, Percent of change from baseline observed in serotonin levels after food and chemical changes. B, Percent of change from baseline observed in levels of total complement (CH-100) after food and chemical challenges. C, Changes in histamine levels from baseline observed after food and chemical challenges. D, Changes in immune complex levels from baseline observed after food and chemical challenges.*

Source: *McGovern, J. J., Lazaroni, J. A., Hicks, M. F., Adler, J. C., and Cleary, P., "Food and Chemical Sensitivity: Clinical and Immunologic Correlates," Archives of Otolaryngology 109:292–297, p. 296 (copyright 1983, American Medical Association).*

patients are more susceptible to foods and chemicals than others. Further, damage by a toxin might compromise detoxification pathways so that other substances formerly metabolized by this pathway could not be degraded properly and thus might provoke symptoms at low exposure levels (a hypothetical basis for the spreading phenomenon).

Levine (1983) has proposed that environmental sensitivities are the result of toxic chemicals reacting with cell constituents to create free radicals (which are formed when a molecule loses an electron). He hypothesizes that if an antioxidant molecule (such as vitamins A, C, E, and selenium) is not present nearby to supply the missing electron, then an electron may be removed from an unsaturated lipid (lipid peroxidation) in a cell membrane, leading to membrane damage, release of prostaglandins and other inflammatory mediators, and formation of antibodies to chemically altered tissue macromolecules.

In 1950, Randolph, collaborating with a surgeon patient of his, Harry G. Clark, published an abstract on the "acid-anoxia-endocrine theory of allergy." Clark, who had food sensitivities, felt that in view of the speed of acute food reactions, changes in electrolytes must be involved (Randolph 1987). Clark knew that allergy was often associated with edema and that one-celled marine organisms swell when acidified; from this he reasoned that because the end products of digestion are acids, perhaps in food-sensitive individuals these acid products of catabolism accumulate intracellularly more rapidly than they can be neutralized by the more alkaline extracellular fluid (including pancreatic bicarbonate). He thus surmised that treatment with alkali salts (that is, bicarbonate salts of sodium and potassium) might be helpful. Indeed, Randolph and Clark found that if alkali salts were administered shortly after an acute food reaction, symptoms were dramatically relieved for many patients. Almost 30 years later, this form of treatment is still used for acute food reactions by clinical ecologists because of its efficacy in many patients. (See further discussion in Chapter 5.)

Vascular Mechanisms

Rea, who began his medical career as a cardiothoracic surgeon, hypothesizes that blood vessel constriction, inflammation, or leakage in multiple organ systems may explain the bizarre combinations of symptoms in these patients. In his view, particular complaints may simply mirror the site and size of affected blood vessels. Spasms in large-caliber arteries, either acutely or chronically, could reduce blood supply to an organ or limb and result in dysfunction, pain, or even necrosis (Rea 1975). Chemical injury to the fragile walls of smaller vessels, however, would be more likely to cause hemorrhage (resulting in petechiae and bruises) or edema

(Rea 1979a). The walls of blood vessels contain smooth muscle. Rea notes that if a patient's symptoms are not explainable by vascular involvement, then other tissues containing smooth muscle such as the respiratory, gastrointestinal, and genitourinary systems are frequently implicated (Rea 1977). Impaired blood vessels or altered smooth muscle function are attractive hypotheses that may explain the diverse and seemingly unrelated symptoms occurring in patients with multiple chemical sensitivities. In the case of either blood vessel or smooth muscle dysfunction, clearly, neurological and immune alterations may play primary roles. A vascular hypothesis might also explain why patients may experience increased pain or other symptoms at the site of an earlier injury or surgery, where blood flow may be relatively compromised.

A final comment regarding the association of food sensitivities with chemical sensitivities is that foods are aggregates of chemicals (Bell 1982; Kammuller et al. 1988), as Table 4-2 demonstrates. The human diet is an important source of exposure to both low- and high-molecular weight compounds. The antibodies to foods that are present in the blood of many individuals attest to the fact that molecules from foods do leave the gut and enter the bloodstream. Thus, any mechanism for the development of sensitivities that might be proposed for chemicals could pertain to foods as well. Butcher and associates (1982) evaluated a worker with TDI sensitivity who could not eat radishes. One bite of a small radish caused severe, immediate bronchoconstriction with a 75 percent decrease in FEV_1, 5 minutes after challenge and necessitated epinephrine treatment. When 26 months later this individual was again able to tolerate isocyanates, he was challenged with 14 grams of radish with no ill effects. The authors note that radishes contain allyl isothiocyanate and benzyl isothiocyanate. However, these chemicals are also present in other foods that the patient was able to eat without adverse effects. This example illustrates a possible connection between sensitivities to environmental chemicals and sensitivity to particular foods. Many similar cases of coexisting food and chemical intolerance have been cited by clinical ecologists. Although their work is often dismissed as "anecdotal," only through observations like these can patterns be discovered, which in turn suggest a hypothesis, which then leads to experiments to prove or disprove that hypothesis. We are currently at the pattern-recognition stage with regard to multiple chemical sensitivities. Finding a mechanism to explain these patterns lies down the road.

TABLE 4-2. Chemical Constituents of Tomato, Apple, Milk, and Orange

Food	Component	Olfactory Threshold (Parts per Billion)
Tomato[a]	Hex-cis-3-enal	0.25
	Deca-trans, trans-2, 4-dienal	0.07
	Dimethylsulfide	0.33
	β-ionone	0.007
	Linalool	6
	Guaiacol	3
	Methyl salicylate	40
	2-Isobutyl thiazole	3.5
Apple[b]	Ethanol	100
	Hexanol	0.5
	Hexanal	0.005
	2-Hexanal	0.017
	Butyl Acetate	0.066
	2-Methylbutylacetate	0.005
	Ethyl 2-methylbutyrate	0.0001
	Hexyl acetate	0.002
Milk[c]	p-Cresol	
	4-Ethylphenol	
	3-n-Propylphenol	
	Phenylacetic acid	
	Hippuric acid	
	Caprylic acid	
	Palmitic acid	
Orange[d]	α-pinene	
	Myrcene	
	Limonene	
	Linalool	
	Cis-2, 8-p-menthadien-l-ol	
	Decanal	
	Carvone	
	Valencene	

[a] From Buttery, R. G., Seilfert, R. M., Guadagni, D. G., and Ling, L. C. Characterization of additional volatile components of tomato. *J Agr Food Chem.* 19(3):524–29, 1971.

[b] From Flath, R. A., Black, D. R., Guadagni, D. G., McFadden, W. H., and Schultz, T. H. Identification and organoleptic evaluation of compounds in Delicious apple sauce. *J Agr Food Chem.* 15(1)29–35, 1967.

[c] From Brewington, C. R., Parks, O. W., and Schwartz, D. P. Conjugated compounds in cow's milk-II. *J Agr Food Chem.* 22:293–94, 1974

[d] From Moshonas, M. G., and Shaw, P. E. Composition of essence oil from overripe oranges. *J Agr Food Chem.* 27(6)1337–39, 1979.

Source: Bell, Iris R., *Clinical Ecology* (Common Knowledge Press, Bolinas, CA, 1982), p. 36.

Possible Psychogenic Mechanisms

Only a decade ago, when news of the first cases of tight building syndrome reached the public, some psychiatrists and psychologists were quick to attribute the subjective complaints of individuals exposed in these buildings to "mass hysteria" or "mass psychogenic illness." In 1979 NIOSH held a symposium entitled "The Diagnosis and Amelioration of Mass Psychogenic Illness," at which one of the authors of this book presented the paper "Mass Psychogenic Illness or Chemically Induced Hypersusceptibility?" (Miller 1979). The presentation was devoted to a discussion of subjective symptoms provoked by exposure to low levels of chemicals, and it sparked a great deal of controversy. The same conference today would more likely be entitled "Indoor Air Pollution" because this phenomenon is now widely recognized. For the most part, mass psychogenic illness has faded from view (Kreiss 1989). However, the possible psychological causes of environmental illness remain a controversial area. To some, the distinction between mind and body is artificial: They are simply two different ways of viewing the same event. In fact, a single process is transpiring. A comprehensive, biopsychosocial approach to patients' problems avoids the pitfalls of reductionistic viewpoints and is thus preferred by many psychologists and psychiatrists (Lipowski 1989).

Two separate issues arise in the context of possible psychiatric origins or contributions to chemical sensitivity. The first relates to the plausibility, nature, and extent of these contributions; the second concerns the most prudent approach toward diagnosis and treatment of the patient when both physiological and psychological factors might be involved. We address the second issue in Chapter 5.

Psychological symptoms are not necessarily psychological in origin. Advances in biological psychiatry focus on genetic and biochemical factors as contributors to central nervous system dysfunction and behavioral disturbance. Environmental exposures can also have psychological sequelae.

The symptoms of low-level chemical exposure may include depression, difficulty concentrating, anxiety, peculiar bodily sensations, headaches, and other subjective symptoms. Patients with multiple chemical sensitivities often report that before they understood what was causing their symptoms they felt as if they could not trust their own bodies or feelings. At any moment, they might feel fine, making plans and commitments for the future; then, the next day or even later the same day, they might feel lethargic, unmotivated, headachy, sleepy, and depressed, as if they had flu. Suddenly, they are unable to fulfill commitments made when they felt energetic. These ups and downs are frequently interpreted by psychiatrists as responses to psychosocial stresses, and patients may be willing to accept such insights because they lack a better explanation. In contrast, patients who have been worked up in an environmental unit often say they are amazed to find direct, clear-cut, cause-and-effect relationships between their symptoms and various foods and chemicals. For the first time, they say they are able to discriminate between their real feelings and those triggered by chemicals. They report that their emotions are appropriate to the situation thereafter, unless, of course, they are having a reaction to a chemical. Not infrequently, such patients feel hostility toward the physicians and psychiatrists who for so long overlooked the chemical basis for their symptoms and instead attributed them to psychiatric causes. These patients wonder how psychiatrists, who routinely use minute doses of chemicals called *drugs* to effectuate behavior, fail to recognize that chemicals in the air or foods can impact the brain or cause marked behavioral changes.

Many of the chemicals these patients implicate as triggering their symptoms are solvents, pesticides, and other substances whose primary target organ, in terms of classical toxicity, is the brain. Interestingly, these individuals who "react" to levels well below those heretofore considered toxic also complain of central nervous system symptoms. Therefore, their complaints are in many respects consistent with known toxic actions of these substances, albeit the *levels* of exposure triggering their reactions are quite different.

Unquestionably, enzymes and various nutrients such as vitamins and minerals act as biological catalysts and regulators. Clearly, any disruption of their function by environmental chemicals might have diverse and far-reaching effects. The limitations of medicine's ability to understand the health complaints of these patients must be honestly and fully acknowledged so that these patients' symptoms are not dismissed as psychiatric when in fact physicians are just beginning to understand the gamut of effects of chemicals on the brain and central nervous system.

Some patients report adverse reactions to particular chemical or food odors, for example, when they smell nail polish remover, cigarette smoke, or popcorn popping. Whether such reactions are classically conditioned responses (Bolla-Wilson 1988) or actual effects of only a few molecules perhaps entrained in the nasopharynx and rapidly transported to the brain is unclear. These responses to odors must be differentiated from those in which mere sight of a food or thought of it produces symptoms.

Researchers at McMaster University in Ontario used classical Pavlovian conditioning to demonstrate that rats sensitized to egg albumen injections in the presence of strobe lights and a humming fan release mediators from their mast cells (IgE mediated) either when injections are given or when the lights and sound are used as the sole stimuli (MacQueen et al. 1989). The authors comment that their results support a role for the nervous system as a regulator of immune function, and they suggest that the nervous system may play a role in colitis, irritable bowel syndrome, and food sensitivities. However, others feel the evidence at present does not support a major role for classical conditioning in human allergic reactions (Metcalfe 1989).

John W. Crayton (1986), a psychiatrist at the University of Chicago, cautions that conditioned responses are more likely to occur in individuals who have true intolerances.

> Undoubtedly, subjects can learn adverse reactions to foods in a classic conditioning sense. However, the presence of these learned reactions may not be helpful in determining whether an individual has "true" adverse reactions to foods. Indeed, it is probably more likely that learned reactions co-exist with true ones. A similar situation occurs in "hysterical epilepsy" in which the patient has gained some conscious or unconscious control over the induction of seizures.

Thus, possible conditioned responses occurring in patients with multiple chemical sensitivities may draw attention away from the true adverse reactions they experience.

That odor conditioning may occur in selected cases is clear. However, patients experience reproducible symptoms to specific chemical exposures (1) often before the odor is perceived (for example, some patients experience symptoms in a particular room or building without detecting an odor, only to learn later that the facility had recently been sprayed with pesticides; Ziem 1989), (2) with their noses clamped during provocative testing, and (3) when anosmia is present (Shim and Williams 1986). These observations weigh heavily against classical conditioning as any more than a partial explanation in certain patients.

It has been suggested that inhaled chemicals may irritate trigeminal free nerve endings in the nose (Doty 1988). Irritation causes a reflexive, involuntary disruption of breathing, a phenomenon familiar to anyone who has inhaled smelling salts. Although trigeminal irritation could explain certain symptoms, such as breathlessness or faintness, in response to pungent olfactory stimuli, it does not explain the entire range of symptoms reported by these patients, often in response to odors that are barely discernible. In addition, patients describe feeling symptoms moments after exposure via intradermal or sublingual routes of administration. Likewise, suppositories placed in contact with mucosal surfaces may provoke onset of symptoms in these patients. Thus, many avenues of exposure may lead to reactions in these patients.

Ecologists observe that patients with chemical sensitivities experience very specific and reproducible constellations of symptoms in response to particular exposures. For example, in one individual, diesel exhaust might trigger sleepiness, mental confusion, and ravenous hunger; rest room deodorizers might be associated with nervousness and irritability; and exposure to a pesticide might be associated with rage followed by uncontrollable crying. Although conditioning could play a role, the fact that responses are *specific* for particular exposures suggests otherwise. Unfortunately, theories of causation that do not fit the reported experiences of these patients, many of whom are highly educated (Doty 1988), abound.

Doty and associates (1988) at the University of Pennsylvania tried to determine whether patients with multiple chemical sensitivities are more sensitive to smells. They exposed 18 patients and 18 healthy control subjects to very low levels (less than 1 percent of permissible occupational levels) of phenyl ethyl alcohol (the principal component of rose oil) and methyl ethyl ketone (a common solvent). Although no difference in ability to detect odors was found between the two groups, nasal resistance was 2 to 3 times higher in the chemically sensitive group than in controls both prior to and following exposure to the odors. Respiratory rates were also higher in subjects than in controls, which the authors felt could be due to nasal constriction because the "nasal airway represents the single largest component of man's total airway resistance and significantly influences tidal volume, respiratory frequency and expiratory time" (Doty 1988). Patients' subjective feelings of not getting enough air or of having labored breathing may reflect increased nasal airway resistance in some patients. Bascom (1990) has noted similar increases in nasal airway resistance among persons claiming sensitivity to tobacco smoke when they are exposed to relatively high concentrations. Doty's patients with chemical sensitivities were no more capable of detecting low-level odors than controls, but they had significantly greater nasal resistances than controls, both at baseline and after challenge. Moreover, 89 percent of the patients had central nervous system symptoms, 67 percent had respiratory symptoms, and 67 percent had gastrointestinal symptoms. At least some of their respiratory symptoms may have been related to their nasal resistance. In addition, these patients had significantly (p <0.005) higher depression scores than did controls.

Urich and co-workers (1988) at the University of Toronto investigated the role of psychological suggestibility in individuals who react to passive smoke. Asthmatics viewed a bank of burning cigarettes during each of their exposures to cigarette smoke but were found not to be particularly suggestible. As the smoke they inhaled increased from zero to moderate to heavy concentrations, there was a progressive dose-response increase in symptoms, deterioration of pulmonary function, increased carboxy-hemoglobin in blood, and increased nasal air flow resistance in subjects that corresponded to exposure levels.

Results of psychological tests also may be misleading in these patients. For example, the Minnesota Multiphasic Personality Inventory (MMPI), a widely used psychological instrument, includes questions concerning peculiar bodily sensations, feelings of inappropriateness, depressed feelings, and many other symptoms, any of which could result from chemical exposures. The chemically sensitive patient who has such symptoms may "read out" as depressed, hypochondriacal, or hysterical on MMPI scales when, in fact, depression, hypochondriasis and hysteria might not be the cause but rather the result of their food and chemical sensitivities.

Food intolerance is a component of several different psychological syndromes involving multiple somatic complaints. Crayton notes over-lapping symptoms among patients diagnosed with neurasthenia, allergic tension fatigue syndrome, and somatoform disorder (Table 4-3), any of whom may complain of food intolerance.

In 1880, Charles Beard published a monograph on neurasthenia that described fatigue, irritability, mental confusion, food intolerances, and numerous other complaints of these patients. He felt diet played an important role and noted that fasting for 4 or 5 days resulted in rapid improvement in some patients. Neurasthenia was regarded (even by Freud) as a predominantly physiological rather than psychological illness (Crayton 1986). The term *neurasthenia,* still commonly used in Europe and the Soviet Union, is no longer favored in the United States. Other diagnostic labels such as *somatization disorder, conversion disorder, dysthymic disorder,* and *neurosis* may be applied to these patients (Crayton 1986).

The diagnostic manual published by the American Psychiatric Association and used by psychiatrists in the United States categorizes a number of disorders characterized by physical complaints under the rubric *somatoform disorder* (DSMIII 1980), which includes somatization disorder, conversion disorder, psychogenic pain disorder, and hypochondriasis.

The syndromes listed in Table 4-3 share many common features. One must wonder whether they might not also share the same etiology, that is, food and chemical incitants. Certainly, the incidence of atopic disorders such as asthma and hay fever is significantly higher among patients with affective disorders (for example, depressives) and their first-degree relatives than among schizophrenics ($p < 0.005$) (Nasr 1981). Undoubtedly, most individuals with food or chemical intolerance who have nasal

TABLE 4-3. Syndromes of Multiple Somatic Complaints

Symptoms	Neurasthenia	Allergic Tension Fatigue	Somatoform Disorder
Fatigue, sickly	+	+	+
Food intolerance	+	+	+
Gastrointestinal symptoms (pain, nausea, vomiting, etc.)	+	+	+
Arthralgias	+	+	+
Myalgias	+	+	+
Cognitive deficits (memory, concentration, etc.)	+	+	+
Palpitations	+	+	+
Insomnia	+	+	0
Headache	+	+	0
Depression	+	+	0
Irritability	+	+	0
Nasal symptoms	0	+	0
Hives	0	+	0
Eczema	0	+	0
Deafness	0	0	+
Blindness	0	0	+
Loss of voice	0	0	+
Convulsions	0	0	+
Sexual indifference	0	0	+

Source: Crayton, J., "Adverse Reactions to Foods: Relevance to Psychiatric Disorders," *Journal of Allergy and Clinical Immunology* (1986) 78(1):243–250, p. 246 (Copyright C. V. Mosby Co., St. Louis).

or skin manifestations would prefer to be seen by an allergist even though they may also experience fatigue, headaches, and memory or concentration problems. Theoretically, different medical specialists such as neurologists, psychiatrists, allergists, gastroenterologists, and rheumatologists may see patients with chemical or food sensitivities in whom varying complaints predominate that drive them to select one specialist over another. Each specialist could be viewing the same problem from a different perspective. Indeed, patients with chemical and food sensitivities may have seen physicians decades ago but were given diagnostic labels such as neurasthenia or the "vapors," an archaic term for a depressive or hysterical neurological condition. Perhaps the latter term will come into vogue again if a chemical etiology for these conditions is affirmed.

A study of 42 patients admitted to the Dallas environmental unit employed a battery of clinical instruments including the MMPI and the Weschler Adult Intelligence Scale–Revised (WAIS-R). Analysis of test results, before and after entering the unit and being on safe foods, showed "statistically significant and clinically meaningful" improvement in five factors: "alienated depression, ineffectiveness, effortful processing, vigilance and effective energy." According to Bertschler et al. (1985), depression lifted, mental acuity improved, feelings of despondency and hopelessness resolved, concentration and short-term memory increased, and energy returned.

Kaye Kilburn (1989a) of the University of Southern California School of Medicine proposes that the human nervous system, because it is so highly evolved, may be most susceptible to environmental agents.

> Sensitivity may be its undoing. The intuitive hypothesis is advanced that the nervous system is the most liable of the body's systems to damage from environmental toxins. Appreciation of damage may be masked because subtle dysfunction is concealed by the nervous system's remarkable redundancy and substitution of functions, or it is overlooked in clinical evaluations which are usually only qualitative.

Physicians who see patients complaining of concentration or memory problems find objective assessment of these complaints difficult. Without careful, quantitative testing and precise knowledge of the patient's abilities prior to the exposure, physicians may erroneously attribute the patient's complaints to anxiety, lack of intelligence, or aging.

A model study of 14 firefighters exposed to polychlorinated biphenyls (PCBs are used to insulate electrical transformers) and their combustion products in a transformer room fire showed significant impairment of memory, cognitive function, and perceptual motor speed compared to unexposed firefighters from the same department (Kilburn 1989). Two days to 3 months after the fire, all 14 of those exposed noted symptoms such as extreme fatigue (8), headaches (7), muscle weakness (9), joint aches (5), memory loss (8), and impaired concentration (6). Only by employing an extensive battery of neurobehavioral tests and comparing scores with controls were their physicians able to detect these alterations, which were very apparent to the firemen themselves. Patients with multiple chemical sensitivities are unlikely to receive such a careful evaluation routinely, nor are preexposure test results or appropriate controls generally available.

Evidence suggests that psychosocial events, such as the death of a spouse or divorce, can suppress immune system function and may predispose certain people to being more sensitive to chemicals at low levels. Certainly, the relationship between psychological and physiological systems is an intricate one.

Selye in his theory of general adaptation and the ecologists both view psychosocial stressors as part of the organism's total stress load. Dantzer and Kelley (1989) review animal and human data suggesting that stress impacts the immune system. The authors caution against the temptation to interpret such data in the context of the psychosomatic model of disease, that is, that one's psychological traits somehow cause immune-related disease via neurological and hormonal correlates. However, because of the feedback loops between the brain and the immune system, an "immunoneuropsychological" interpretation may be closer to the biological truth. Presumably, undetectable changes in the immune system may alter central nervous system function and produce psychological and emotional manifestations. For example, in the early stages of cancer, products released by immune or tumor cells may produce the helpless, hopeless feelings that have been associated with progression of the disease.

Analogously many of the psychological and emotional problems experienced by patients with multiple chemical sensitivities may be the result of currently undetectable alterations in their immune or nervous systems, rather than the result of personality problems or a belief system.

Two of the most vocal critics of clinical ecology, allergists John Selner and Abba Terr, are of the opinion that multiple chemical sensitivity patients adhere to a "belief system" that chemicals are the cause of their health problems. Staudenmayer and Selner (1987) describe what they term "an irrational belief system":

> The ecology belief system usually is deeply entrenched and its logic well developed by intricate rationalizations and indoctrination. Social factors feed on the primary and secondary gain of the victim. "True believers" are more than willing to present their testimonials, seeking and affording mutual assurance. The social and psychological dynamics of the cult apply. In addition, there exists a plethora of "health publications" that provide the authority of print, while an impulsive media, eager for news, often is duped by unsubstantiated and unscientific claims of so-called ecology authorities.

Terr (1989c) believes that no psychotherapeutic intervention will help these patients, whereas Selner (1988, p. 51) advocates systematic deprogramming of the patients to purge them of their beliefs and believes that 50 to 75 percent of receptive patients can be deprogrammed. Staudenmayer and Selner emphasize that those patients with chemical sensitivity who adhere to a belief system, particularly so-called universal reactors, must be separated from those who are truly sensitive to specific, identifiable chemicals.

Some psychiatrists strongly feel that individuals with multiple chemi-

or combinations of these (Schottenfeld 1987; Brodsky 1987). According to Schottenfeld (1987), "the early childhood history of individuals with M.C.S. [Multiple Chemical Sensitivities] is often notable for the presence of physical or sexual abuse, severe medical illness during childhood, death of one or both parents, or other severe disturbances of early caregiving relationships."

According to Staudenmayer (1989), at first many patients will not reveal problems of childhood abuse, but when trust is established in a therapeutic relationship, they will. Whether persons with chemical sensitivities experience as youths more psychological trauma than the "average" has not been determined. Knowing what percentage of "normal" individuals undergoing the same degree of intensive psychological inquiry would confess to similar difficulties is important. Otherwise, this particular approach to the problem suffers from the same flaws the clinical ecologists have been accused of with regard to study design.

Staudenmayer and Selner (1990) compared 58 patients with multiple chemical sensitivity, 89 patients from a psychology practice (diagnoses included depression, anxiety, mood swings, phobia, panic, and insomnia), and 55 controls reported not to have had psychological symptoms for at least one year (diagnoses included asthma, gastrointestinal problems, headaches, skin problems, hypertension, and menstrual pain). All patients underwent a battery of neuropsychophysiologic tests. Electroencephalograms (EEGs) for the psychology patients and for the multiple chemical sensitivity patients differed significantly from those of the controls ($p < 0.001$). However, the authors conclude that "the universal reactor group was not statistically different from the psychologic group" ($p = 0.22$). Patients with multiple chemical sensitivity had significantly higher scalp electromyographic (EMG) activity than did the other groups ($p < 0.001$ in both cases). The authors felt their data confirmed their hypotheses "that the group of universal reactors would not be significantly different from a group of outpatients with overt psychologic disorder who did not project them onto the environment" and "that universal reactors manifest psychosomatic illness rather than true environmental disease." While these hypotheses could explain their data, their psychology practice population might also have chemical sensitivities, accounting for the similarities in EEGs. The statistically significant difference in EMGs suggests real differences between universal reactors and psychologic patients. Unfortunately, this study does little to clarify the etiology of multiple chemical sensitivity. In a published critique, Davidoff et al. (1991) also question the authors' interpretation of their data and suggest that "Psychological and psychiatric disturbances could simply be consequences, rather than causes, of MCS [Multiple Chemical Sensitivities]."

Even if chemically sensitive patients have had more early trauma, two other questions must be asked. First, could major psychological trauma somehow predispose individuals to developing bona fide sensitivities to chemicals? Ecology patients sometimes report a major life event coincided with the onset of their difficulties; however, such life changes are frequently associated with changes in *exposures,* for example, a move to a different home following a divorce or spouse's death, or taking medications during stressful times. Consider chemical sensitivities that might arise during exposures from remodeling that could be manifested as irritability or depression. If a divorce ensues, the development of chemical sensitivities might be attributed to the "stress" of the divorce, when in fact the sensitivities may have contributed to both the stress and the divorce. Staudenmayer and Selner (1987; 1990) assert that they have performed blinded chemical testing using sham challenges as controls with patients who claim to have this condition and that these challenges result in both false positives and false negatives. In their view, these alleged erroneous reactions by patients confirm the lack of true sensitivities and provide a point of departure for the psychologist to explore with patients their "belief system" about having chemical sensitivities. In examining the experimental design for these challenges, crucial questions that have not yet been addressed in published studies are:

1. Are subjects in a deadapted state prior to the challenge so that extraneous exposures during and prior to the challenge (up to several days before) do not interfere with testing?

2. Are open challenges performed first to confirm that the placebo (a masking odor such as peppermint) is in fact a placebo and that the "active" challenge is something to which the patient has had demonstrable reactions?

3. What is the recency and latency of the patient's exposure to the substance being tested? In other words, has enough time elapsed (about a week or so) that the person is no longer adapted or reacting to the last exposure but not so much time that the sensitivity has waned? Recency of exposure is recognized as a crucial variable in conducting challenges in patients with occupational asthma, for example.

Finally, with regard to the issue of childhood abuse or childhood illness, one must ask whether the parents and families of chemically sensitive patients (patients who often have psychological manifestations) might not also have such problems. Ecologists suggest some genetic predisposition to this problem. Abusive or alcoholic parents of chemically sensitive patients may have suffered from unrecognized environmental sensitivities themselves (see the appendix regarding alcoholism and drug abuse and neurobehavioral and psychiatric manifestations).

Ecologists argue that major illness during childhood may have been the result of undiagnosed chemical sensitivities or that sensitivities may have been triggered by infection or medications that were administered, rather than viewing these events as a disruption in the care-giving relationship or the beginnings of secondary gain, that is, seeking attention or nurturing via illness. Therefore, even if one could prove that childhood trauma were more prevalent among patients, such a finding neither proves psychological interpretations nor disproves chemical causes.

Schottenfeld (1987) offers advice to physicians who work with these patients: "Regardless of the original etiology of symptoms, these individuals tend to amplify their symptoms and to develop the mistaken belief that the symptoms are indicative of severe disease."

> Changes in the workplace that reduce toxic exposure and the risk of exposure may provide the most reassurance—the installation of a new exhaust system in Mrs. A.'s workplace was an extremely effective psychotherapeutic intervention in addition to its obvious benefit in the prevention of occupational respiratory disease (Schottenfeld 1987).

Another psychiatrist (Brodsky 1987) writes:

> A review of medical history and literature that reflects on medical cultures reveals that there have always been people who have had unpleasant physical and emotional symptoms and experiences for which they sought explanations. . . . In the culture of 20th century medicine, a disorder of the immune system would represent a sophisticated and acceptable explanation, because the immune system is demonstrably complex and is inter-related with all other systems, and no one would disagree that many of its mechanisms and manifestations are still unknown.

Recently, Black et al. (1990) reported that 15 of 23 subjects (65%) diagnosed with environmental illness by clinical ecologists had at one time met the criteria for a mood, anxiety or somatoform disorder versus 13 of 46 matched healthy controls (28%). These authors conclude that such patients may have one or more commonly recognized psychiatric conditions that could explain some or all of their symptoms. Critics of Black's study draw attention to the fact that more than a third of the patients claiming environmental illness had no history of significant psychopathology in their lifetimes, therefore mental illness did not explain ther problems (Galland 1991) The study was further criticized for failing to consider that individuals who have quit working or been hospitlaized for *any* illness will exhibit more psychological symptomatology than healthy controls (Galland 1991). Black responds that while he believes that psychiatric conditons may explain most, or all, symptoms in some individuals, he suspects that other patients diagnosed as having environmentsl illness may have a "verifiable physical disorder that would explain their symptoms equally well" (Black 1991).

The issue of whether chemical sensitivity is a bona fide physical entity, or, an "irrational belief system" that may be "systematically deprogrammed," or a form of psychopathology amenable to psychotherapudic interventions is a critical one, one that merits thoughtful consideration and rigorous scientific iquiry.

The issue of whether chemical sensitivity is a bona fide and potentially widespread problem or, rather, an "irrational belief system" held by fewer individuals who may be "systematically deprogrammed" is a critical one, one that merits thoughtful consideration and rigorous scientific inquiry.

Conclusions

Perhaps the mechanism for multiple chemical sensitivities is not identifiable; that is, after all avenues of biochemical and immunological inquiry have been exhausted, no single explanation for this disorder is forthcoming. The theory of substance-specific adaptation is based upon observations of the responses of patients in a deadapted state who are worked up in an environmental unit. Adaptation is *only* an observation at this time, not a mechanism. However, biological *limits* might regulate how much an organism can adapt, limits that could be highly individual and vary by orders of magnitude. Certainly adaptation occurs at all levels of biological systems, from enzyme systems to cells, tissues, organs, and even behavior (Fregly 1969). Theoretically, a major insult or the accumulation of lower-level injuries within these systems could lead to a kind of "overload" or "saturation" effect with respect to adaptive capacity that would cause an individual to have environmental responses, which, instead of being flexible and fluid, are now fragile and overly responsive. Many patients we interviewed for this book told us that even years and in some cases decades following the onset of their problems they had recovered only a portion of their former energies and tolerance for their environment. Their descriptions seem to suggest the loss of an intangible capacity to adapt, parts of which may be temporary and recoverable and other parts of which may not. We are reminded here of the teaching: "Listen to the patient. He is telling you the diagnosis." Perhaps they are telling us the mechanism as well.

CHAPTER 5

Diagnosis and Treatment

Diagnostic Approaches

As with most fields in medicine, meticulous history taking is the most important element in making a diagnosis. However, history taking for multiple chemical sensitivities involves obtaining a chronology not only of illness but of exposures as well. "Although the physical examination is an integral part of all medical investigation, 'examination of the environment' of a patient tends to be relatively more rewarding" (Randolph 1987, p. 274). Physicians today must ask their patients what kind of work they do and inquire about specific chemical exposures on and off the job and changes in symptoms at work, on weekends, and during vacations. Ramazzini, the father of occupational medicine, instructed physicians to ask, "Of what trade are you?" On the whole, occupational health practitioners today, more than other medical specialists, take the most comprehensive exposure histories. Thus, for patients who may have multiple chemical sensitivities resulting from industrial, tight building, or community exposures, the physician group most attuned to and therefore likely to discover the potential link between the patient's illness and a chemical exposure is the occupational physician. The "new generation" of occupational health physicians is well informed about chemicals, various processes, and associated exposures, as well as signs and symptoms resulting from chemical exposure (Rosenstock 1984). They are familiar with the industrial hygienists' measurements of chemical exposure. However, before they can help chemically sensitive patients, they will require instruction in the particular symptoms, provoking exposures, and special problems of these patients. Occupational health physicians and clinical ecologists have overlapping interests and would benefit from information exchange and cross-training. Likewise, allergists, by learning more about chemicals and toxicology as recommended by some of their spokesmen (Selner and Staudenmayer 1985b; Bardana and Montanaro 1989) and by taking exposure histories that go beyond the confines of IgE-mediated disease, could emerge as a major physician group specializing in the problems of these patients in the future.

An adequate exposure history with attention given to pinpointing when symptoms began in relation to other factors (for example, drugs, chemical exposures, job changes, household moves, operations and hobbies) is essential. Concurrent illness in other household members, co-workers, and even pets may provide clues. This time-consuming detective work is the *sine qua non* for discovering an inciting exposure. Properly designed patient questionnaires may facilitate the process by enabling the patient to engage in the detective work as well. Questions concerning the patients' likes or dislikes for certain odors may be revealing because aversion to particular odors has been noted commonly among patients who have multiple chemical sensitivities (Randolph 1980). Over the years, Randolph has noted that the more odors checked off on his questionnaire as "strongly like" or "strongly dislike," the more likely the patient is to have chemical sensitivities. In addition, patients can prepare a chronology or time line of major events such as household moves, job changes, surgeries, and pregnancies and the onset and duration of symptoms or illness. Similarly, a daily log of activities or exposures that notes any symptoms may facilitate recognition of patterns.

Of course, the more symptoms and the more systems of the body affected, especially the nervous system, and the more these symptoms fluctuate in intensity, the stronger should be the physician's suspicion of multiple chemical sensitivities. Johnson and Rea (1989) report that the average patient entering the Dallas environmental unit has five symptom complaints, many of which are neurological. Industrial workers with multiple chemical sensitivities exhibit similar constellations of symptoms (Cone et al. 1987). A history of multiple "idiosyncratic" drug reactions or alcohol or food intolerance or cravings may also be suggestive (see Chapter 3).

The physical exam, traditionally an important diagnostic tool, disappointingly is often normal in these patients. Symptoms or signs may occur only with exposure. Injury may be subclinical and prepathological. Laboratory findings may be normal or, if abnormal, provide no pattern or clue that seems to have clinical relevance. Altered helper-suppressor T-lymphocyte ratios and the presence of autoimmune anti-bodies may be suggestive (see Chapter 4), but are not diagnostic. Subtle signs of vasculitis can be noted in some; spontaneous bruising, pete-chiae, and cold or blue extremities (Raynaud's phenomenon) may occur.

Rea has noted yellowish skin discoloration with normal liver function tests in some patients and refers to this as the "chemical yellows." Al-lergic shiners (dark circles under the eyes, or "racoon eyes," from renous congestion), Dennie's lines (creases under the eyes), reddening of the ears, and the "allergic salute" (nose rubbing) might provide clues in some children (Rapp and Bamberg 1986); these facial features are rec-ognized by allergists in children with both classical IgE-mediated allergy and nonallergic, non-IgE rhinitis (etiology of the latter is unknown but conceivably could be related to food or chemical exposures).

Rea and associates are exploring more sophisticated and objective ways of measuring changes in their patients, such as monitoring sym-pathetic and parasympathetic nervous system activity by recording pu-pillary reactions to a light stimulus (discussed in Chapter 4) and using a balance recorder, a platform on which the patient stands and attempts to maintain balance. Movements of the patient are recorded and reflect disturbances in one or more of the three physiological inputs that regu-late balance: visual input, the inner ear, and proprioceptive signals. PET (positron emission tomography) or other brain-scanning techniques may prove helpful in the future (Morrow 1990).

As discussed in detail in Chapter 2, the gold standard for diagnosing chemical hyperreactivity in a patient is the environmental unit, coupled with fasting. Although this approach may be too costly and time-con-suming for the average patient, for the very ill, it may be the *only* way to unravel this multifactorial, polysymptomatic illness. Eventually, biom-arkers may be developed for chemical sensitivity, especially if the mech-anisms of the disease are biochemical or immunological. However, if the nervous or limbic system is key, it may not be possible to identify biom-arkers.

Short of a several-week stay in an environmental unit, might any other approach be used to diagnose chemical and food sensitivities in patients who do not require hospitalization or who may wish to be worked up as outpatients? Certainly an elimination diet could be attempted to identify food incitants. Patients may have difficulty fasting or avoiding common incitants, rotating their foods, or obtaining chemically less contaminated foods. (Even so-called organic foods may not be entirely free of pesti-cides and other contaminants.) Detecting subtle chemical sensitivities while at home could be quite difficult. Masking or adaptation to chemicals in one's home environment (such as gas furnace emissions) might go unrecognized. If comprehensive environmental control were attempted at home, major remodeling or overhauling of furniture, heating systems, wardrobe, and other major changes may be required in order to achieve a chemically less contaminated environment for the patient. Such interventions done in a hit-or-miss fashion could be costly. Far better would be residences that are relatively "safe" habitats, such as specially constructed trailers or homes in which patients could reside temporarily while they sort out their sensitivities and undergo food and chemical testing. We inspected trailers lined with porcelain that have been specially made for chemically sensitive individuals and visited a small community outside Dallas, where specially constructed homes are occupied by chemically sensitive patients.

Clearly, the cost and trouble of such a rigorous diagnostic approach may be prohibitive for the average patient with chemical sensitivities. For this reason, provocation-neutralization has been promoted by ecologists as a way to diagnose and treat at least some of their patients' sensitivities to biological inhalants, foods, and chemicals. This procedure is considered in detail in the next section, which discusses therapies. Less widely accepted and far more controversial diagnostic approaches used by the minority of clinical ecologists include electroacupuncture and kinesiology . The basis for these procedures is speculative at best; they are not addressed in this book.

Therapies

To the traditional practitioner, perhaps the most disturbing feature of clinical ecology is the wide range of therapeutic modalities used by various practitioners and the lack of proof for many of them. Many allergists with whom we spoke expressed frustration with an attitude among certain clinical ecologists that they do not need science because they are right. Allergists are critical of clinical ecology's lack of randomized, double-blind clinical trials. Randolph (1987, p. 220) and other ecologists feel this criticism is "overdrawn." They emphasize the clinical nature of the field: its concepts and techniques are inductively derived from careful clinical observation. As rigorous and cautious as Randolph's use of an environmental unit might have been, the same cannot be said for other treatment approaches used by clinical ecologists. We discuss here some of the more frequently used ecologists' therapies, including provocation-neutralization, nutritional supplementation, detoxification, and the treatment of acute reactions to foods and chemicals. Fundamentally, clinical ecologists agree that avoidance of incitants, both food and chemical, is the treatment of choice and allows the best possibility for recovery. Clearly, however, this treatment is not entirely satisfactory.

Avoidance can lead to an ascetic life-style that is unacceptable to many patients. Some who are very ill feel they have no choice. A number of treatment modalities have been employed by ecologists in an attempt to speed their patients' recoveries; however, no study has been done to demonstrate whether patients receiving these treatments recuperated any faster than if they had practiced avoidance alone.

Provocation-Neutralization

The majority of clinical ecologists use provocation-neutralization to a greater or lesser extent. This technique involves provoking a patient's symptoms by injecting under the skin or administering sublingually a small dose of an inhalant, food, or chemical while observing the patient for symptoms and/or increase in wheal size if given via a cutaneous route. This diagnostic test is used to identify incitants for a particular patient. Subsequently, various dilutions of the same substance that produced symptoms or a wheal are injected or given sublingually until one dilution is found that turns off the patient's symptoms or that results in no increase in wheal size following intradermal injection. This dose is called the *neutralizing* dose.

A lengthy review of all studies of provocation-neutralization done to date is beyond the scope of this book. Further, we feel strongly that too much emphasis has been placed upon trying to disprove this method as if the existence of the problem of multiple chemical sensitivities depended on provocation-neutralization. The existence of multiple chemical sensitivities and the efficacy of provocation-neutralization are independent issues and ought to be treated as such.

Suffice it to say that provocation-neutralization may be an evolving technique, just as classical allergy testing is still evolving. Salvaggio, an allergist, has remarked upon the paucity of evidence to support the efficacy of mold immunotherapy that is used by classical allergists (Salvaggio and Aukrust 1981). Others offer similar views:

> Immunotherapy has been used empirically over the past 70 years, primarily because the actual immunologic mechanism has continued to elude investigators (Gurka and Rocklin 1988).

> The mechanisms by which hyposensitization is achieved are not completely understood. . . . While statistically controlled blinded studies on the efficacy of allergens and immunotherapy have been made, for the most part, only for some pollens, extension of these results to other allergens and certain conditions is generally considered acceptable (package insert from an allergenic extract).

Immunotherapy was used by allergists for decades before the discovery of IgE by Ishizaka in 1969. Controlled trials demonstrating its effectiveness have been available only since the 1950s. Van Metre and Adkinson (1988, p. 1329) describe the difficulties faced by investigators who wish to design controlled trials for testing the efficacy of immunotherapy:

> Design requirements are complex and difficult to accomplish in any one single trial. These difficulties can be addressed by developing a model of specific aeroallergen disease with which multiple groups of investigators can work over a relatively long period of time. Methods and reagents are refined until consistent, accurate results are achieved.

Such trials are difficult and costly to conduct. Large, *homogeneous* groups of patients must be recruited, for example, a large number of patients with seasonal hay fever triggered by ragweed pollen. Here each patient has the same symptom resulting from the same exposure. The added complexity of multiple symptoms resulting from many divergent exposures (as occurs in multiple chemical sensitivities) is obvious. The same authors recognize that trials using provocation-neutralization have had major problems with reproducibility, nonstandardized extracts, nonhomogeneous patient populations, and disparate methods of measuring outcome; yet they comment favorably on studies by Boris and others (1985a; see also Boris et al. 1988) using provocation-neutralization in two randomized, placebo-controlled, double-blind, crossover studies for cat and dog extract causing asthma and state that "the work deserves careful study and attempts at replication." Their comments contrast sharply with the position paper by the American Academy of Allergy (1981) on this subject: "Subcutaneous provocation and neutralization as a method for the treatment and diagnosis of allergic disease has no plausible rationale or immunologic basis."

A recent and comprehensive study of provocation-neutralization was supported by the American Academy of Otolaryngic Allergists (AAOA) and reported in *Otolaryngology: Head and Neck Surgery*, a leading ENT journal. Approximately 1,800 members of AAOA use these methods, which are endorsed by the 8,000 members of the American Academy of Otolaryngology Head and Neck Surgery, the largest group of ENT physicians in the country. William King and co-workers' studies (1988a, 1988b, 1989), sponsored by the AAOA, reported that provocation-neutralization had a sensitivity of 79.7 percent and a specificity of 72.4 percent, in contrast to classical skin testing, which had a sensitivity of only 26.6 percent and specificity of 85.5 percent when compared with a provocative food challenge. In his 1986 presidential address to the

American Academy of Allergy and Immunology, John Salvaggio (1986) referred to " 'fringe element' societies such as the otolaryngologists' allergy society, in which unproven methods of immunodiagnosis and therapy are used." Otolaryngologists who practice provocation-neutralization are not appreciative of the organized write-in campaigns by allergists that have successfully persuaded the Health Care Financing Administration to deny payment for provocation-neutralization for foods. Some merely regard these campaigns by the allergists as a turf battle between the allergists and clinical ecologists.

Sublingual provocation and neutralization is used much less often than injection techniques. Blinding is more difficult for sublingual provocation than for injection. Moreover, many ecologists feel that the clinical result is not as good. Nevertheless, sublingual testing and treatment have high patient acceptance and low risk of adverse reactions. Recent sublingual treatment studies using house dust mite (Scadding and Brostoff 1986) show promise for this approach. Many think the venous network beneath the tongue is responsible for uptake of foreign substances, and research using animals points toward a more direct pathway from the oropharynx to the brain (for example, the hypothalamus) involving very rapid substance transport (Kare 1968; Maller et al. 1967). Such a mechanism might help to explain the rapid alterations in mental status patients report with provocation and neutralization by the oral route, as well as the rapid onset of symptoms they experience when ingesting or inhaling incitants.

The definitive study of provocation-neutralization has not yet been done, and the studies purporting to prove its ineffectiveness have not been free from substantial flaws. Most convincing are individual cases in which symptoms appear dramatically with provocation (Miller 1977; Rapp 1978a, 1978b). The technique may work best in a select subgroup of patients. Indeed, the collective strength of the dozen or so positive studies done to date may be greater than that of any individual study; the statistical technique of meta-analysis may have relevance here as a tool for evaluating them further (Louis et al. 1985; Wachter 1988).

David King, University of California, San Francisco, (1984, 1988) has carefully reviewed studies of provocation-neutralization, and his work is important reading for anyone wishing to understand this subject. He reviews two of the studies upon which the American Academy of Allergy and Immunology relied for its position statement against provocative testing. One was a study by Caplin (1973) sponsored by the American College of Allergists. King (1984) renanalyzes Caplin's data and finds that the reported statistical analysis was incorrect. In fact, the validity coefficient *is* significant, implying that results of provocation *were* related to results of feeding challenges. Similarly, King examines a study by

Lehman (1980) that reported that sublingual testing was not reliable. Lehman did not analyze the data statistically to reach this conclusion. King found that the testing was in fact reliable for two of the four foods tested, even though a very restrictive dependent measure was used for evaluation (nasal mucosal changes for which the reliability of the experimenter's judgment was unknown). King (1984) concludes: "A close examination of other frequently cited evaluation studies reveals similar flaws, making firm conclusions about provocative testing premature." In another paper King (1988) reviews other studies that have found provocative testing unreliable or invalid, including the often cited study by Jewett et al. (1990). In their study three "active" and nine placebo intradermal injections were administered to 18 clinical ecology patients by clinical ecologists. Only patients who consistently had symptoms provoked during open challenges were studied. Small doses ("underdoses") of food injections were administered double-blind, and the subjects guessed which were active and which were placebo. The results of guessing by subjects were no better than chance. Prior to its publication King raised several important concerns about the Jewett study.

1. Patients may have been avoiding the food in question and thus have lost their prior sensitivity (see Chapter 2 regarding adaptation).
2. The use of an either-or, dichotomous measure (guessing active or placebo) coupled with single-subject data analysis will detect only relatively strong effects and may work only for a highly accurate test, not one prone to a certain amount of error.
3. Possibly underdoses are ineffective, and larger doses may provoke reactions in some patients.

King (1981) himself conducted a study of provocation testing and found that allergenic extracts under double-blind conditions could provoke cognitive-emotional symptoms in selected individuals. However, his enthusiasm for provocation-neutralization is carefully tempered. He notes that symptoms are frequently reported by subjects given placebos, "a finding which should concern clinicians employing the test" (D. King 1988). Conceivably, the high rate of placebo reactions may reflect background fluctuation in chronic masked reactions to a less than optimal test environment and suggest the need for trials to be conducted in a controlled, less chemically contaminated environment. King concludes:

> Most studies of provocative food testing contain serious flaws which limit inferences regarding reliability and validity. Thus, whether these tests are sufficiently reliable and valid for clinical use cannot, strictly speaking, be determined from the research available, since the appro-

priately designed studies have not yet been conducted. However, the research that has been reviewed would seem to suggest that both [intradermal and sublingual] methods of testing can provoke symptoms above placebo levels, but that these effects are generally quite small. Such subtle effects, when combined with symptoms that naturally vary over time and with placebo effects, would make it unlikely that their use in the clinical setting is as accurate as some proponents claim. On the other hand, the data do not support the conclusion that these methods cannot provoke genuine symptoms. Rather, the problem is distinguishing the "signal" from the noise. Averaging across many trials, as in group research, aids this process, but this fact is of little use in the clinic, in which every individual test is interpreted.

King's reservations concerning the clinical utility of provocation-neutralization are crucial. Although provocation-neutralization may be in the beginning stages of its evolution, much like traditional allergy immunotherapy was earlier this century, its continued use should depend on objective demonstration of efficacy. Patients should not be held hostage by controversies in this area. With so few available therapies, those that may offer benefits should not be barred but investigated further. Both otolaryngologists and ecologists realize there are limitations to provocation-neutralization's effectiveness. Rea (1989), who probably sees the most severe patients, finds that 30 to 40 percent of patients are *not* helped by provocation-neutralization techniques but feels that its failures should not preclude its use in the 60 to 70 percent who may receive benefit. Most clinical ecologists continue to stress the importance of avoidance as the primary and most efficacious treatment with concomitant use of a rotary diet, but acknowledge compliance may be difficult for many patients.

We asked several ecologists whether, by using neutralizing doses on a frequent basis, one might not simply be masking patients' symptoms, that is, inducing adaptation that might obscure chronic damage caused by administering incitants on a regular schedule. They were concerned over this point, but most discerned a big difference between a patient's taking neutralizing doses on a daily basis and a patient's eating the food on a daily basis. They argue that the former generally would not result in symptoms, whereas actual food ingestion would.

Even if provocation-neutralization were proven valid, extension of this technique from inhalants and foods to chemicals such as formaldehyde, automobile exhaust, phenol, and tobacco smoke is a major leap of faith that needs much further investigation. Exposing patients to levels of chemicals normally encountered in everyday life may be justifiable. However, injection of potentially carcinogenic substances such as formaldehyde or auto exhaust is of concern. Ecologists argue that their patients normally are exposed to these substances at even higher doses, and low doses will not increase risk to any measurable degree.

If provocation-neutralization were to be established as efficacious in clinical trials, evaluation of its long-term efficacy (the longest trials have been on the order of a few weeks) versus avoidance alone would be a next, important step.

A further consideration with regard to provocation-neutralization is that the background level of pollutants in the testing room or those brought in on patients' clothing or skin (such as traffic exhaust or cigarette smoke) might interfere with accurate provocation and/or neutralization. In addition, the time interval since the patient was last exposed to the test substance may affect the provoking and neutralizing doses, just as an individual's response to ozone or other substances may be affected greatly by recency of exposure (see Chapter 2). Thus, adaptation or acclimatization must be considered as a potentially important, if not crucial, variable. If the testing room where provocation-neutralization is being done contains volatile organic compounds, cause-and-effect relationships could be obscured. At present, we have no reason to suppose that skin testing or sublingual testing would be any different in this respect from oral or inhalation challenges conducted in an environmental unit. Background levels and the time interval since the last exposure to a substance must be rigorously addressed in any future studies.

To some, the most convincing bits of evidence in favor of provocation-neutralization come from the many anecdotal cases reported by ecologists. Doris Rapp has filmed several such cases using double-blind procedures. Nevertheless, traditional allergists raise concerns about appropriate control of conditions and her objectivity. Some discount her work by implying that the adults must be acting and the children either hungry or in need of a nap. We wonder whether these anecdotal cases, in which reactions to foods or chemicals seem to be turned on or off by a tiny amount of incitant, might not represent individuals whose sensitivity is very high and thus the reaction is easily observed. If so, these individuals may present a unique opportunity to study and document this phenomenon. Provocations in these individuals must be done with sufficient iterations to satisfy statistical requirements, as was attempted by Jewett et al. (1990). Again, the effect of background noise on the testing must be assessed because inadvertent exposures (food or chemical) could interfere with test results. Perhaps such testing is most sensitive and specific if performed on patients in the deadapted state in an environmental unit where background noise is negligible. A further difficulty, reported by a number of patients, is a tendency for their "endpoints" to shift over time, which may lead to an increase in their symptoms. Although their physicians might recommend retesting, many simply discontinue treatment when this occurs.

Detoxification

The EPA, in its ongoing program to monitor levels of toxic chemicals in human adipose tissue, has found many volatile organic compounds and pesticides in all parts of the body, including the brain and nervous system. Some of these chemicals may persist for decades; for example, beginning in 1973, Michigan residents were exposed to PBB (polybrominated biphenyl) a toxic fire retardant that accidentally had been substituted for a nutritional supplement in farm animals (Wolff et al. 1982). A clinical research team from Mount Sinai School of Medicine found that 97 percent of more than 1,000 state residents had detectable PBB in their fat (0.2 ppb or more). Because serum levels taken 12 to 18 months apart in 1977 and 1978 from the same individuals were not significantly different, the researchers concluded that the PBB in their tissues would remain there indefinitely (Wolff et al. 1979).

A detoxification method employing sauna, exercise, polyunsaturated oils, and various nutrients that has been used in the field of drug rehabilitation for drug accumulations in fatty tissue was offered to seven healthy male volunteers from Michigan. Following the detoxification regimen, fat biopsies from these individuals showed significant reductions in 16 chemicals (averaging 21.3 percent reduction), including PBB. Four months later, after no further treatment, the same subjects nonetheless had additional decreases in chemical fat stores: the average decrease in the 16 chemicals studied was 42.4 percent. Schnare of the EPA et al. (1984) hypothesized that this continued decline might suggest recovery of the body's own ability to eliminate toxic substances. Others have reported use of detoxification therapy for toxicity subsequent to exposure to dioxin (Roehm 1983), PCBs and their by-products (Schnare 1986; Tretjak 1989; Kilburn 1989), and other chemicals (Root 1987). Specifically, the detoxification regimen involves seven components (Schnare et al. 1982):

1. Aerobic exercise for 20 to 30 minutes to increase fat mobilization
2. Low temperature sauna (140–180° F) for 2 or more hours (preferably 5 hours) after exercise to enhance skin excretion of toxic substances
3. Nutritional supplements with gradually increasing amounts of niacin to enhance lipolysis, and proportionate amounts of other vitamins and minerals

4. Water, salt, and potassium replacement
5. Polyunsaturated oil, 2 to 8 tablespoons a day as tolerated, to decrease uptake of toxins in the intestine and facilitate their excretion
6. Calcium and magnesium supplements
7. A daily routine of exercise and sauna for a period of several weeks, balanced meals, adequate rest, and no drugs, alcohol, or medications

This approach is not considered a cure but is claimed to facilitate the recovery of certain patients with multiple chemical sensitivities. Randolph (1980) cites several cases in which significant improvements in patients' food and chemical sensitivities have occurred and states:

> The task of defining the relationship between exogenous and endogenous chemicals in particular patients remains. At this time, we can say that reducing endogenous accumulations of toxic chemicals appears vitally important to the effective treatment of some environmentally ill patients; and the development of a safe and effective method for reducing these burdens gives us a welcome new tool for treatment.

A study of 14 firemen exposed to PCBs in a transformer room fire employed an extensive battery of neurobehavioral tests that was administered 6 months after the fire and again 6 weeks later after the exposed firemen underwent a 2- to 3-week sauna detoxification program (Kilburn 1989b). Controls were firemen from the same department not exposed to the PCB fire. The 14 exposed firefighters showed impaired short-term memory, interpretation of designs, spatial relationship integration, decision-making, and coordination. Following detoxification, cognitive function and memory improved significantly ($p < 0.05$), but other measures did not. Nevertheless, the subjects' own perception of their difficulties did not improve. The effectiveness of detoxification could not be determined conclusively, and the authors urged caution in attributing improvement to detoxification. Serum and body fat PCB content before detoxification did not correlate with results of neurobehavioral tests. The PCB levels were not repeated after detoxification. Thermal decomposition of PCBs, as occurs in a fire, yields polychlorinated dibenzofurans and dioxins that may be 100 to 10,000 times more toxic than PCBs. The authors comment that tissue levels of these byproducts, if they could be measured, might correlate better with symptoms and neurobehavioral indices. Clearly, such trials need to be replicated. The mass balance of chemicals must be tracked carefully to be sure that chemicals are not migrating to other parts of the body and that they are being excreted.

Xylene, a solvent that off-gases from paints, varnishes, glues, printing inks, and other sources, is one of the most prevalent indoor air contaminants. Riihimaki and Savolainen (1980) exposed healthy male volunteers to constant (100 or 200 ppm) and varying (200 or 400 ppm hourly peaks) concentrations of xylene, adjusting baseline concentrations in the latter case so that a mean concentration of 100 or 200 ppm was maintained. Exposures occurred over a six-hour period (with a one-hour break at noon) for five days, followed by a two-day weekend and one to three more days of active exposure to xylene. A variety of psychophysiologic parameters were measured, including reaction time, body balance, manual dexterity, and nystagmus. Following cessation of exposure, breath xylene concentrations fell rapidly at first (half-life about 0.5 to 1.0 hours) during the first few hours after which the elimination rate slowed markedly (half-life about 20 to 30 hours). Elimination from fat was estimated to be even slower, around a half-life of 58 hours. Indeed after six days of exposure (5 days + weekend + 1 day), the concentration of xylene in gluteal subcutaneous fat was ten times higher than the blood concentration at the end of the last day of exposure. Thus some accumulation of xylene in fat occurs over several weeks of repeated daily exposure. The data underscore the potential importance of a detoxification method that would accelerate the elimination process. Indeed, elimination of xylene from the body is relatively rapid compared to many xenobiotics whose half-lives are on the order of weeks, months, and years. Most indoor air contaminants are solvents whose tissue levels will be minimal (though from a health standpoint still potentially significant) after several days' avoidance of exposure. In future studies it will be important to document changes in blood levels and tissue levels of target substances, such as xylene, in those who enter an environmental unit or undergo sauna detoxification.

Of particular interest, Riihimaki and Savolainen (1980) observed that most of the adverse effects of xylene upon their normal subjects "tended to disappear after a few succeeding days of exposure." However, "after the weekend away from exposure, the effects were again discernible." They conclude: "This phenomenon suggests that tolerance had developed over a few days with regard to psychophysiological effects by xylene." Parallel to this, the authors observed that fluctuating (as opposed to continuous) concentrations of xylene provoked EEG changes consistent with decreased vigilance. In one subject who had had a normal EEG when he entered the study, fluctuating xylene concentrations provoked bilateral spike and wave complexes suggestive of marked interference with brain electrical activity. Thus exposures occurring minutes or even days before testing may influence the response to a test reexposure. Adaptation, which figures prominently in responses to xylene and ozone, likely affects responses to other xenobiotics. Avoidance of exposure (by having patients change residences or jobs or by utilizing an environmental unit) begins the process of deadaptation. Clearly, finding some way to hasten this process would be helpful, particularly during the late, slow phases of elimination of chemicals from bodystores, for example, from adipose tissue. For this reason, sauna detoxification, if effective and safe, might prove an attractive treatment alternative.

Nutritional Approaches

Extensive data now indicate that vitamins and minerals influence the toxicity of environmental incitants. Amino acids and fat content of the diet also may be important. For example, vitamin E deficiency increases ozone toxicity in rats. An awareness of the role of nutrition in allergy is also developing. Low vitamin B_6 concentrations have been found in adult asthmatics, and supplementation with B_6 produced a dramatic drop in the frequency and severity of wheezing or asthma attacks (Reynolds and Natta 1985). Another recent paper reports significant improvement in atopic dermatitis with vitamin C supplementation (Kline et al. 1989).

Rea and other clinical ecologists (Johnson and Rea 1989; Rogers 1990) routinely measure vitamin and mineral levels in their patients with chemical sensitivities and supplement as indicated. In a sample of 118 patients studied in the environmental control unit in Dallas, mineral levels outside the normal range were found in 53 percent (higher than normal) of the patients for magnesium, 88 percent (lower than normal) for chromium, and 47 percent (higher than normal) for aluminum (Johnson and Rea 1989). A number of abnormal vitamin levels were also found. In some cases. testing for deficiencies involves more than a routine blood test; Rea feels that red blood cell and plasma magnesium levels are poor indicators and prefers an intravenous magnesium challenge to assess magnesium status (Rea et al. 1986b). When ecologists recommend nutritional supplements for their patients, most exercise extreme caution to avoid vitamins derived from food sources that might trigger symptoms; for example, vitamin C from sago palm may be substituted for the usual commercial vitamin C preparations, which often contain corn. McLellan (1987) cautions that before nutritional therapies are embraced too quickly, one must recognize the lack of human data and the fact that most available research pertains to the interaction between single nutrients and single toxins in relatively high doses in contrast to the mixed exposures at lower levels encountered by the patient with multiple chemical sensitivities. However, nutritional status is relatively easy to measure, supplementation can be done fairly safely, and at least a theoretical basis exists for using supplements. Animal and human research have supported use of antioxidants, vitamins A, C, and E, and selenium to protect against certain pollutants (Calabrese 1978; Shakman 1974). Such antioxidants may prevent free radical production that could trigger synthesis of inflammatory prostaglandins (Metz 1981; Cross 1987). Levine (1983) advocates use of antioxidants such as vitamins A, C, and E, zinc, and selenium to prevent free radical formation, which can result in cell membrane damage, release of inflammatory mediators, and perhaps formation of antibodies to altered tissue macromolecules.

Galland (1987) reports several nutritional abnormalities, most notably decreased excretion of essential amino acids in 40 percent of his chemically sensitive patients despite a high-protein diet. Erythrocyte superoxide dismutase activity was decreased in 89 percent (24 patients) versus 79 percent (15) in allergic controls (not significant); erythrocyte glutathione peroxidase activity was decreased in 48 percent (11) versus 36 percent (5) allergic controls (not significant). Some of Galland's controls might have been misclassified because all had either allergies or somatic complaints such as fatigue. Nevertheless, Galland reports that supplementation with antioxidants, including selenium, copper, zinc, and sulfur-containing amino acids, produced major clinical improvement in 25 percent (14) of chemically sensitive patients.

An enormous number of other therapies too numerous to mention have been invoked by clinical ecologists and others. These include dietary, neutralization, and pharmaceutical treatments for candidiasis (indeed, some *traditional* allergists mentioned they found nystatin beneficial in treating certain patients for systemic candidiasis, and they wished for more data to help evaluate this treatment), acupuncture, pancreatic enzymes for food intolerance, oral sodium cromoglycate for food intolerance, and transfer factor. These therapies are outside the scope of this book, but clearly a host of therapies, many of which have been severely criticized for being "unproven," are being offered to patients with multiple chemical sensitivities in an effort to improve their outcome. Some patients report that they obtain small increments of benefit, occasionally more, from each intervention, but none is curative.

For the patient who is having an acute reaction to an environmental incitant or food, ecologists recommend certain "first aid" treatments. In the event of an acute reaction, particularly to a food, some patients take baking soda or a combination of sodium bicarbonate, potassium bicarbonate, and calcium carbonate (so-called tri-salts) with water. They claim these measures relieve their symptoms within moments. Critics caution against possible dangers in using such treatments indiscriminately, for example, as the treatment for IgE-mediated food anaphylaxis. The ecologists' rationale for this therapy, which patients claim can be quite effective acutely, was discussed in Chapter 4. Some use powdered vitamin C mixed in water to mitigate a reaction. In severe cases, for example, to stop a seizure resulting from a food or chemical challenge, some ecologists administer bicarbonate or vitamin C intravenously. Administration of oxygen has also been used in severe reactions. Randolph (1987, pp. 50–51) examined scleral blood vessels of patients before, during, and after reactions to foods and noted increased sludging of red cells; he reasoned that such clumps decreased the red blood cells' ability to carry oxygen. Others have criticized the use of oxygen in these patients without first obtaining a blood oxygen level (Terr 1986). However, oxygen is accepted by many as an effective drug for certain medical conditions, even if the blood oxygen level is normal. The manner in which these treatments are administered to patients is likewise important. Plastic or rubber face masks and fresh plastic tubing commonly used for oxygen and intravenous lines may leach small amounts of plasticizers or other substances and provoke severe symptoms in some chemically sensitive patients.

In summary, clinical ecologists employ a wide variety of treatments, some unproven, in their efforts to help their chemically sensitive patients. When first used, any medical therapy is experimental, but because placebo effects may be significant, ultimately careful, blinded clinical trials are essential for establishing a therapy's value. Increasingly, it is argued that patients with disabling diseases demand and deserve the opportunity to try new, albeit unproven, treatments, provided these do not result in serious harm. Few medical therapies are without some hazard: over the past 39 years, at least 46 deaths have occured following conventional allergy shots or skin testing (Lockey 1987).

Arguments concerning ecological therapies must be kept in perspective. Salvaggio, an allergist, reflected upon the role of unproven therapies in medicine (Salvaggio and Aukrust 1981):

> The practice of medicine will, to be sure, remain primarily an art rather than a science, and physicians will of necessity continue to use clinical judgment and weigh benefit/risk ratios in prescribing a large number of therapeutic procedures that have not been proved to be efficacious by controlled studies. Indeed, one could fill several pages with a list of commonly employed therapeutic procedures in all fields of medicine that have not been proved to be efficacious.

Psychological Interventions

The discussion in Chapter 4 on possible psychogenic mechanisms argues that chemical sensitivity may have physiological causes, psychogenic causes, or both. The search for a cause in a specific patient is most likely to lead a physician to pursue one avenue before investigating the other. Often, however, only one avenue is pursued. The investigator or diagnostician could make either of two kinds of mistakes: in pursuit of an environmental cause, true psychogenic causes could be ignored or, alternatively, in pursuit of a psychogenic cause, true environmental causes could be ignored. The consequences of making those mistakes are different. Pursuing the psychiatric route first may subject the patient to the complexities of establishing a therapeutic relationship and/or the prescribing of psychoactive drugs, and both may generate doubts concerning the patient's mental health. In addition, psychotherapy may be unproductive if environmental causes are at work. Labeling a patient as having a psychiatric illness may be pejorative from the perspective of an employer, co-workers, and family. That psychiatric records are kept separate from the medical records of patients is no accident. In the event that psychoactive drugs are used, unraveling an environmental cause or contribution to the patient's underlying condition may be greatly complicated.

Alternatively, if environmental causes of the illness are investigated first, especially with double-blind, placebo-controlled study in an environmental unit, the patient may discover an environmental cause; even if the patient does not, the confidence or justification with which a psychogenic etiology could be pursued is strengthened. Workup in an environmental unit is unlikely to interfere with or complicate subsequent psychiatric workup, and thus a mistake made in choosing this option (investigating environmental causes first) can be more easily remedied. Black et al. (1990) and Rosenberg et al. (1990) suggest approaches which physicians who are skeptical about the existence of chemical sensitivity may employ to help establish a therapeutic relationship and keep their patients "within the medical fold" (Black 1990). Galland (1990) argues "One cannot empower a patient and at the same time dismiss his or her puzzling symptoms as psychogenic." Black acknowledges that the patients he studied who had seen clinical ecologists were generally satisfied with their ecologist and dissatisfied withe the approaches of traditional medicine. Ecologists offered support and understanding of their pain and suffering and a physical explanation for their symptoms.

When adequate controlled studies are done, it may be revealed that some or even the majority of individuals with multiple chemical sensitivities have had episodes of depression or other psychological symptoms years prior to the onset of major disability. For example, Simon et al. (1990) report that plastics workers who developed environmental illness were more likely than controls to have a prior history of anxiety or depression (54 percent versus 4 percent) and a larger number of medically unexplained illnesses (6.2 versus 2.9). It bears repeating that prior psychiatric symptomatology neither proves a psychogenic etiology nor disproves an environmental one. Patients who are disabled by multiple chemical sensitivities may represent a more sensitive subset of the population because of their genetic endowment or even exposures as children. Members of this group may experience depression, asthma, or headaches at low levels of chemical exposure for years without being aware of the cause, yet after a major exposure they might become disabled and exhibit greatly magnified sensitivities to subsequent low level exposures. Thus the persons most likely to develop multiple chemical sensitivities may in fact be those who were more sensitive to begin with, though not recognized as such.

In summary, one can remain agnostic about which route is likely to uncover the truth regarding causation, but the costs of erring are significantly different regarding the two routes of investigation. We think that these facts are sufficiently compelling to justify the investigation of environmental causes first, before committing patients to potentially detrimental psychiatric interventions, such as long-term psychodynamic psychotherapy or long-term medication. Certain short-term or focused cognitive or behavioral therapies may be beneficial but should not be relied on to the exclusion of evaluating the chemical component. Once diagnosed, chemically sensitive patients may find psychotherapy, biofeedback, and other approaches supportive while they make lifestyle changes.

Areas of Agreement and Disagreement between Allergists and Clinical Ecologists

On the basis of interviews with key individuals in allergy, clinical ecology, and occupational medicine, as well as the literature we reviewed, we have discovered both areas of common ground regarding the chemically sensitive patient and areas of disagreement. Although some of the tension between allergists and clinical ecologists may stem from a competition for patients, the differences in their scientific and medical viewpoints are also more fundamental. All physicians agree that chemical exposure can be harmful to any and all systems of the body. Disagreements exist as to what levels of exposure are necessary to cause health effects, what particular symptoms or diseases are associated with specific chemical exposures, and what mechanisms of causation come into play. The range of opinion is wide as to the extent to which the problems of the chemically sensitive patient are psychogenic in origin.

Physicians we interviewed concurred that isolation of the patient in an appropriate environmental unit away from chemical substances in food, air, and water is essential to unraveling the myriad substances that may be causing a variety of effects. More specifically, all of the traditional allergists with whom we spoke acknowledged that in the study or workup of patients with possible environmentally induced disease attention must be paid to the potential role of adaptation. Low-level exposure to chemicals must be avoided prior to testing patients for chemical sensitivities in order to avoid adaptation and the loss of a measurable effect. All allergists acknowledged the necessity of controlling for adaptation in any rigorous study of chemical sensitivity, as has been done in the study of ozone (see Chapter 2). Further, all agreed that an environmental unit such as that formerly operated by Dr. Selner in Denver would be an important tool for future investigation and understanding of chemical sensitivities.

Some allergists tend to favor psychiatric referral for patients who do not improve, whereas clinical ecologists are of the opinion that patients' problems, although difficult to solve, are nonetheless likely to be physical in nature. Ecologists feel that environmental factors must be carefully excluded (in an environmental unit if necessary) prior to invoking psychiatric diagnoses.

All physicians agree on the need for studies to clarify unproven therapies, and some physicians in both allergy and clinical ecology think both specialties ought to work together to design the necessary protocols, conduct the studies, and evaluate the results. A few allergists are embracing the fundamentals of clinical ecology such as adaptation and avoidance, but decline to identify their views with those of the clinical ecologists. Allergists have been openly hostile to clinical ecology in the past (AAAI 1980, 1981, 1986). Recently, however, some physicians have become tired of name-calling and legal entanglement, which they recognize as contrary to their patients' best interests, and increasingly want to air and resolve their differences and identify avenues of cooperation. For a fuller understanding of the differences in viewpoints between allergists and clinical ecologists, see Bell's (1987b) article and Terr's position paper on clinical ecology for the American College of Physicians (1989).

PART · III

Responding to the Problem

CHAPTER 6

Needs, Concerns, and Recommendations

Research Needs

> The time has come to give to the study of the responses that the living organism makes to its environment the same dignity and support which is being given at present to the study of the component parts of the organism. . . . Exclusive emphasis on the reductionist approach will otherwise lead biology and medicine into blind alleys.
>
> René Dubos

Earlier chapters of this book focused on the magnitude and nature of the chemical sensitivity problem, possible mechanisms, diagnostic approaches, and therapies. These chapters addressed various issues from the perspective of an individual patient or, perhaps more correctly, from the perspective of a physician-scientist looking at individual patients. A problem with such a variety of possible causes and multitude of possible effects might seem to be hopelessly complex to sort out, but in a very real sense the complexity and multifactorial nature of the problem may contribute to its clarification.

Patients with chemical sensitivity differ among themselves and present themselves differently to different physicians. The diagnosis patients receive appears to depend in a very real sense upon which physician's door they enter. Moreover, very different people enter particular

147

physician's doors, manifesting a referral and selection bias. For example, Rea sees individual referrals from other physicians and self-referred patients, 20 percent of whom go on disability, whereas Terr published data on patients referred to him for evaluation, mostly for compensation purposes. Physicians seeing patients with problems stemming from tight buildings or industrial workplaces may see still different groups of affected individuals. The proverbial problem of the blind men and the elephant is the result.

An important research goal is not only the accurate characterization of symptoms and their relationship to specific chemicals but, more fundamentally, characterization of the various populations or groups that appear to be chemically sensitive. We have attempted a preliminary categorization in Table 6-1. Refinement of this categorization is essential and must be the first step in sorting out the myriad chemically caused sensitivities, some of which may represent classical toxicity, some classical allergy, and some what we term multiple chemical sensitivities. Of special importance is the identification of sensitizing events, when they occur.

The four rather distinct groups of patients are: industrial workers; workers and schoolchildren in tight buildings; members of communities exposed to air and water pollution from toxic waste dumps, aerial pesticide spraying, groundwater contamination, or other industrial exposures; and a heterogeneous collection of individuals whose exposure may come from domestic indoor air, consumer products, pesticide use, or other personal contact.

As the description of the patient demographics in Table 6-1 reveals, these patients often may differ greatly in employment or professional characteristics, socioeconomic status, sex, and age. They are also likely to see very different categories of physicians. Industrial workers are much more likely to see occupational physicians or private physicians; the sickest workers may eventually consult clinical ecologists. Individuals suffering from sick building syndrome are not as likely to seek out or be referred to clinical ecologists, even though they are conscious of the fact that their problems stem from tight buildings. People in polluted communities may find themselves going from physician to physician before seeing a clinical ecologist who then may determine that their problems are related to chemicals; by the time these individuals see the clinical ecologist, they may be frustrated, angry, and confused. Finally, the host of other individuals whose exposure to chemicals comes from domestic indoor air, consumer products, pesticide use, and the like may vary greatly in the type and the seriousness of their symptoms and are likely to have seen a series of physicians including allergists and clinical ecologists. The most difficult patients encountered by the clinical ecologists and some allergists may ultimately be referred to Rea, who often sees those most seriously afflicted, persons whose condition therefore may be less reversible. He also probably sees a greater diversity of persons with chemical sensitivities than are represented in the other three groups discussed above. In contrast, those allergists who see chemically sensitive patients referred for worker's compensation evaluation may view only a small segment of the most ill patients.

Multiple chemical sensitivities thus encompass a broad spectrum of people. The allergist sees them either because the patients believe they have an "allergy" or because they are referred by insurance companies or employers for workers' compensation purposes. Which physicians see which patients seems to affect greatly the acceptability of their problem as a bona fide physical illness, or at least not a problem of psychogenic origin. Relatively few physicians today would call hypochondriacal those who are affected by tight buildings. Most workers with chemical sensitivities seek workers' compensation as a matter of last resort. They would prefer to be able to work (Davis 1989).

The exposure-patient profile of people suffering from chemical sensitivities has to be characterized accurately in order to fashion an appropriate response. Such a categorization may also be useful in suggesting areas of research that might be undertaken by federal agencies such as the National Institute for Occupational Safety and Health (NIOSH), the National Institute of Environmental Health Sciences (NIEHS), the Environmental Protection Agency (EPA), and the Agency for Toxic Substances and Disease Registry (ATSDR), which is concerned especially with community-based pollution related to toxic waste facilities and contamination of water supplies and has cooperative agreements with 11 states to undertake surveillance studies in contaminated communities for exposure and disease. In addition, state-based efforts, usually involving state departments of health and possibly state departments of environmental protection, need to be encouraged. In the event that the federal government is not willing to undertake research as to both the nature and the etiologies of chemical sensitivity disorders, a multistate effort may well be advisable.

Most scientific criticisms of clinical ecology have been directed toward the efficacy of provocation-neutralization therapies. To focus initial research efforts in this area would be of limited value because most traditional practitioners question the diagnosis itself. Clinical ecologists must continue to develop objective means of measuring symptoms and relating them to exposures.

A properly constructed environmental health unit could serve as a focal point for studying chemically sensitive patients in the deadapted or unmasked state. Allergists, clinical ecologists, and toxicologists should

TABLE 6-1. Spectrum of Multiple Chemical Sensitivities

Aspects	Industrial Exposure	Tight Buildings
Recognition of problem	Workers themselves; unions; occupational health clinics	Office or school workers themselves; parents of school children; school nurses
Place of diagnosis	Occupational health clinic; private physician's office	Private physician's office; occupational health clinic
Nature of exposure	Industrial chemicals; acute or chronic exposure	Off-gassing from construction materials, office equipment, or supplies; tobacco smoke; inadequate ventilation
Demographics; awareness	Primarily males, blue-collar, 20s to 60s; conscious of classical workplace hazards; often aware of relationship between symptoms and exposure (e.g., better on weekends/vacations, worse at times of peak production or during certain processes, etc.). Awareness via word of mouth, union, occupational physician	Females more than males; children; white-collar office workers and professionals; 20s to 60s; aware of symptoms associated with change in building environment, e.g., new construction, carpeting or seasonal illness. Awareness via word of mouth, media, field study
Manifestations	Multiple symptoms involving multiple systems with marked variability in type and degree of symptoms. CNS symptoms common. Physical exam most often unremarkable	Multiple symptoms involving multiple systems with marked variability in type and degree of symptoms. CNS symptoms common. Physical exam most often unremarkable. Many have symptoms of eye, nose, throat irritation, and malaise
Average severity of illness or disability[a] (varies greatly with individual)	Moderate to severe	Mild

[a] Those individuals whose symptoms are most persistent and disabling often see a series of physicians before they finally see an ecologist. Rea's clinic represents a kind of tertiary referral system for ecologists who send him the most severe cases. Thus the patients Rea sees are markedly different, i.e., more disabled, than the typical patient seen by an allergist.

Community-based Air and Water Pollution	Individual Exposures
Individuals in community; government-sponsored field surveys	Individuals themselves
Private physician's office; state-supported clinical study	Private physician's office
Toxic waste dumps, aerial pesticide spraying, ground water contamination, air contamination by nearby industry, and other community exposures	Heterogeneous, personal; indoor air (domestic), consumer products, pesticide use
All ages, males and females; children/infants may be affected first/most; middle to lower class; community awareness via word of mouth, community action groups, media, or field study	70–80% females; 50% in 30-to-50 age bracket (Johnson 1989); white; middle class, upper middle class, and professionals; awareness via word of mouth, patient groups, physicians
Multiple symptoms involving multiple systems with marked variability in type and degree of symptoms. CNS symptoms common. Physical exam most often unremarkable.	Multiple symptoms involving multiple systems with marked variability in type and degree of symptoms. CNS symptoms common. Physical exam most often unremarkable.
Mild to moderate	Mild to moderate if referred to allergists or clinical ecologists. Severe if seen by Rea in Dallas. Disabling if admitted to environmental unit or an applicant for workers' compensation or disability.

contribute to the design of any such study to ensure acceptance of the results. The unit should be constructed and operated following the highest academic standards. For reasons discussed in Chapter 1, epidemiological studies on chemically sensitive populations have to be designed with extreme care, or no evidence will emerge at statistically significant levels. The study group must be appropriately defined, and more than one symptom may need to be counted as a health effect. Biomarkers of both sensitization and sensitivity should be identified, when possible. If immunologic or biochemical mechanisms are involved, this may be a promising area; biomarkers involving the limbic or nervous system in general, however, may be more difficult, if not impossible, to identify, especially since there may not be a blood-borne marker.

Given clinical ecology's low status and reputation in the scientific community at the present time, independent researchers have serious disincentives to examine its tenets. Yet a critical and unbiased airing of the problem of chemical sensitivities is needed. All aspects of the problem —from documentation of the sensitivity itself to diagnostic approaches for its discovery to the range of possible therapies—need attention. The National Academy of Science Panel on the Interrelationships of Toxic Exposures and Immune Response should be encouraged to study the problems of multiple chemical sensitivities as well as problems of immune system damage or dysfunction.

Government and university scientists must be allowed and even encouraged (by grants) to participate in research in this field without being hamstrung by the opinions of traditional medical practitioners. Science is not served by continuing to deny the probable existence of the problem in the face of massive and growing circumstantial evidence, although admittedly subjective in many respects. A better approach would be to acknowledge that something appears to be going on, that low levels of chemicals can affect the body in subtle ways that currently escape our understanding, and that individual susceptibility to environmental agents may vary by several orders of magnitude.

The widely circulated journals representing traditional medicine must also allow unbiased airing of this problem, as they have with other issues, for example, medical versus surgical treatment of coronary artery disease. Numerous university and government scientists who are knowledgeable about chemical sensitivity feel it is worth taking seriously. However, many fear for their own professional careers and are reluctant to write or speak openly on the subject. Fortunately, this appears to be changing. Debate rather than unilateral criticisms of unproven ideas is what is needed to encourage defensible research on these ideas. Certainly, criticisms of therapies should not be used to foster a denial of the existence of chemical sensitivity altogether. Recently, physicians and scientists appear to be more willing to accept the concept of chemical sensitivity in the context of occupational exposures or tight buildings. Perhaps because most patients suffering from these exposures do not seek clinical ecologists, mainstream physicians are probably more accepting of the problems in those contexts. If clinical ecologists are involved, there seems to be more of a desire to shoot the messenger than to take the problem seriously. As similarities are recognized among patients whose exposures arise in different contexts, we hope a more scrutinizing evaluation will be forthcoming.

Patient and Community Concerns

In this section we articulate the concerns and needs of the chemically sensitive patient and the needs of the community in preventing illness triggered by or associated with low-level exposures to chemicals. These needs include information; health care; alternative schooling, employment, and housing; medical insurance; compensation for disability; social and legal services; and the control of chemicals in the office, industrial workplace, home, and consumer products.

Information

Information about Chemical Sensitivity.   Chemically sensitive persons need information and guidance concerning the recognition of chemical sensitivity and the availability of diagnostic tools and possibly effective therapies. They need to understand that chemicals can cause both classically recognized environmental and occupational disease (such as lead or solvent poisoning or allergic reactions to organic dust) and less understood, but nonetheless real, problems associated with low-level exposures. Industrial workplaces can give rise to both kinds of environmental illness, and unraveling the vagaries of causation there may be especially difficult. Home and office environments also present a mixture of illnesses, perhaps more often characterized by lower exposure levels. Episodic exposures to chemicals present still different challenges. Chemically sensitive persons need assistance in understanding their condition so that they can make reasoned choices about the health care or preventive actions they might pursue.

Information about Chemicals.   Chemically sensitive patients need to know the potential hazards of the chemicals they work with or may be exposed to. Federal and state right-to-know legislation and the Superfund

Amendments and Reauthorization Act (SARA) Title III reporting requirements are important legal avenues for information held by government agencies, employers, and manufacturers and producers. However, patients may need more specific information that perhaps could be provided by industrial hygiene surveys by OSHA, state agencies, or possibly insurance carriers. Access for individuals to state and federal sources for information and services is needed.

Health Care

Access to Appropriate Care from Private Physicians and Clinics.   In one profile of chemically sensitive patients seen at a clinical ecology clinic, 30 percent of the patients had seen six to ten physicians before coming to the unit (Johnson and Rea 1989). Brodsky (1987, p. 695) observes:

> Many of these patients shift from one specialist to another, going from family physicians to allergists to neurologists and other medical specialists, and to chiropractors, acupuncturists, homeopaths, and even faith healers. Both the patients and their physicians feel frustrated and dissatisfied, the patients because they remain convinced that their symptoms signal a physical disorder for which a medical explanation must exist and the physicians because they have been impotent as healers, unable to help these obviously distressed individuals or to reassure them that they do not have a serious disease. Such patients are time-consuming and in clinic settings not infrequently objects of derision.

Our investigations make clear that the chemically sensitive patient finds medical care by trial and error and by word of mouth. A more directed path and identification of helpful physicians and clinics are needed. Patients whose problems stem from occupational, sick building, or home environments may each need different care, as might persons suffering from episodic exposures. No sensible referral system exists, and the segmented nature of medical care and the inability of some physicians to acknowledge a disease they do not understand contribute to the personal suffering of the sometimes bewildered patient. Multispecialty clinics, health maintenance organizations (HMOs), and preferred provider organizations (PPOs) unfortunately rarely include specialists in diseases caused by chemicals. Occupational medicine clinics have the potential for expanding their concerns and services into illnesses caused by low-level exposures, but specific initiatives are needed to bring about this expansion. Taking work and/or environmental histories is essential to delivering appropriate medical care. Industrial hygiene services in both the home and workplace may also be indispensable.

University-based clinics, such as that at the Robert Wood Johnson Medical School in New Jersey, have the potential for rapidly incorporating new knowledge and perspectives more quickly for the recognition, diagnosis, and treatment of the chemically sensitive patient. The potential needs to be realized, however.

Avoidance. The first line of defense for the chemically sensitive patient is avoidance of offending chemicals and substances found or suspected to cause problems. Some kinds of avoidance are easy, but others are very difficult. Persons suffering from sick building illness may have to abandon employment or residence in those buildings. Some new EPA offices have been planned, which have windows that open, no carpeting, no copier machines, and other features, in an effort to accommodate sensitive employees. In the case of children who are chemically sensitive, an alternative to home tutoring may be the state provision of environmentally safe classrooms where students with documented and suspected chemically related disorders could be educated and observed for follow-up. This practice is currently being pursued in Canada (Rapp and Bamberg 1986). In Maryland's guidelines for indoor air quality in schools, modification of workplace exposure limits is recommended (Maryland 1987, p. 6).

Alternative Employment and Housing

Alternative Employment. Federal and state laws require that employers provide handicapped workers reasonable accommodation. Deciding whether a chemically sensitive person is handicapped is done on a case-by-case basis. In some instances, work at home may be possible; the EPA seems to have reached this accommodation with some of its chemically sensitive employees (Hirzy 1989b). Patients who are not considered handicapped nonetheless need rehabilitation and return to gainful employment.

Alternative Housing. Some chemically sensitive patients cannot live in their prior domiciles. Because of severe economic consequences, some assistance is obviously needed. Options include halfway houses for the severely affected and the establishment of experimental communities in less polluted areas.

Medical Insurance

Receiving reimbursement for medical expenses incurred when the diagnosis and treatment of chemical sensitivity is performed by clinical ecologists is becoming increasingly difficult (Davis 1989). Even though a prominent allergist and critic of clinical ecology, Abba Terr (1989b) has stated that "what we do is as unproven as some of the things we are criticizing," allergists have organized letter-writing campaigns to urge the Health Care Financing Administration (HCFA) to deny reimbursement for "unproven" techniques. Such efforts do not seem to deter the desperate patient from seeking medical care; they just make the patient more desperate. Recognition of diagnosis and treatment of chemical sensitivity for insurance purposes is necessary on grounds of fairness and, in the case of some patients, to enable them to receive adequate care. For traditional medical practitioners to throw up their hands and not be able to help these patients and, at the same time, to lobby vigorously to deny them therapies that sometimes, if not often, relieve their suffering cannot be justified.

Compensation

Chemically sensitive patients are sometimes unable to continue in a specific workplace, often an industrial workplace, or may not be able to work at all. Workers' compensation systems have been painfully slow to provide coverage for occupational diseases. Employers and their insurance carriers have historically denied the work-relatedness of disease associated with chemical exposures; for example, 60 percent of occupational lung disease claims are contested (U.S. Department of Labor 1980). Compensation for the chemically sensitive worker is vigorously resisted, and in some cases patients have to be labeled with a psychiatric disorder such as posttraumatic stress disorder in order to receive compensation for their illness. Earon Davis (1989), an attorney and executive editor of the *Ecological Illness Law Report* believes that only about 1 percent of severely affected chemically sensitive workers will file a workers' compensation claim because they do not want to be labeled as psychiatric cases. In addition, many workers leave jobs because of chemical sensitivity only to find themselves unable to tolerate a new job and unable to file a claim against either the new or old employer.

In most instances chemically sensitive people cannot trace their problems to a specific work-related exposure and may seek disability payments under Social Security. William Rea (1989), who sees the most severely affected patients, reports that about 20 percent of those he sees go on disability. In cases of illness stemming from pesticide exposure or from some other episodic exposure involving industrial or consumer products, the patient may seek compensation through a suit in tort. In 1987, the Consumer and Victims Coalition Committee of the Trial Lawyers of America adopted a resolution supporting "environmental illness" victims. Recovery of damages based on alleged immune system damage is becoming more commonplace, and the manufacturers and insurance industry are reacting vigorously. Dennis Connolly (1988), an insurance executive, writes:

> Courts as well as scientists are routinely grappling with the problems of harmfulness and causation. A disturbing trend from the point of view of those who might be looking toward providing insurance is the increased use of various forms of marginal science to overcome difficulties in proving causation. "Clinical ecology" is a "science" offering broad support for causation in bodily injury cases, but the science has been repudiated by many in the medical establishment and cited as an example of poor science flourishing in the courtroom.

Academics who have joined the criticism include Donald Elliott (1988), who writes that "plantiffs in toxic tort cases are increasingly relying on testimony by a small group of professional witnesses called 'clinical ecologists' (whose views are repudiated by the scientific establishment). Lay juries and the public are vulnerable to being misled by such 'experts.' "

A more thoughtful analysis of the use of clinical ecology in the courts is provided by Sheila Jasanoff. After tracing the successes and failures of patients in their attempts to establish harm to their immune system by using the testimony of clinical ecologists, Jasanoff (1989, pp. 86–87) notes: "That medical societies [the American Academy of Allergy and Immunology and the California Medical Association] might not be wholly disinterested in their efforts to discredit a competing, and apparently successful, specialty does not seem to have been a worry [to the court]." She concludes that these societies "proved effective because these organizations defined the boundaries of valid medical science in a way that courts could not readily ignore." Nonetheless, the principles established by clinical ecology are enjoying some success in the courts (Cornfeld 1989).

Powerful economic and industrial forces have joined to deny the chemically sensitive patient compensation, just as they did earlier in this century for occupational injury and later for occupational disease, by accusing the worker of malingering and bad faith. The issue of compensation may seem peripheral to the scientific-medical debate over chemical sensitivity, but it is actually central to the resolution of public policy in this area. Economic issues heighten the conflicts between allergists and clinical ecologists and need to be resolved if an optimum scientific consensus is to be achieved. The existence or origins of the patients' disease are contested in conflicts over who should pay while the patient continues to suffer. Brodsky (1987, p. 696) observes: "Private and public agencies that provide disability benefits argue that these patients are not truly disabled, although those dealing with them recognize that they are in great distress."

Social and Legal Services

As with others debilitated by disease, chemically sensitive people need psychological, financial, and legal counseling to enable them to manage their affairs, seek help from appropriate government agencies, and cope with stress. Some of these services can be provided by state government and private patient-support groups. Earon Davis (1989) reports that many chemically sensitive persons suffer neuropsychological defects often resulting from continuing unavoidable exposures and have extreme difficulty interfacing with the legal or social service systems. He argues that these persons need social workers, not lawyers, who can guide them into avenues that improve their situation. Such guidance could be provided at halfway houses or special communities.

The Regulation of Chemical Exposures and Other Preventive Initiatives

The community has an interest in preventing and limiting the problems of chemical sensitivity. For chemical sensitivity that has its origin in exposures to chemicals in the workplace, pesticides, chemical spills, and the like, adherence to and enforcement of *existing* environmental regulations is necessary to prevent sensitization of more individuals. The existing standards of OSHA, EPA, and state agencies do not, however, protect those individuals already sensitized. New regulations governing inadequately regulated substances or unregulated applications of chemicals, such as pesticides or other chemicals applied in office buildings, schools, or apartment complexes, are also needed. (Following health complaints associated with new carpeting at EPA headquarters in Washington, D.C., the EPA union petitioned EPA to regulate 4-phenylcyclohexene, the chemical suspected of causing health problems [National Federation of Federal Employees 1989]. However, the EPA denied the petition and instead embarked on a program involving voluntary testing of all carpet-related volatile chemicals by carpet companies [EPA 1990].) At a minimum, regulators should require that application of chemicals, such as pesticides, be accompanied by adequate notice so that people can avoid the exposure. Currently most OSHA and EPA regulations control exposures at the parts per million (ppm) level. More stringent regulations may be needed to protect both sensitized (and hence chemically sensitive) individuals and those who may become sensitized. The mandates behind environmental regulation do indeed require the protection of sensitive populations (Friedman 1981). If regulations are imposed to *prevent sensitization*, it may be less necessary to control exposure more stringently in the future in order to *control sensitivity*, because people will not be sensitized in the first place.

The appearance of similar kinds of health problems in widely divergent populations exposed to chemicals (see Table 1-1) illustrates that the failure to regulate adequately or prevent exposures to chemicals in the environment, workplace, and consumer products has resulted in the present chemically sensitive population. In order to protect this population from further or continuing damage, some chemicals, such as formaldehyde, will need to be controlled at the part per billion (ppb) range or banned outright for some uses (Massachusetts 1989, pp. 74–102). Although the regulation of chemicals traditionally has been viewed as a federal government initiative with states as secondary partners, states may have to take vigorous regulatory action in order to protect the chemically sensitive. Massachusetts, for example, banned the use of urea formaldehyde foam insulation. California regulated vinyl chloride levels in ambient air, even though the federal government issued only emission limitations. Other states may need to examine the adequacy of their regulations.

The Role of Medical Practitioners and Their Societies

The roles that primary care physicians, occupational and environmental health physicians, allergists, and clinical ecologists can play in addressing the needs of the chemically sensitive patient differ, depending upon the group of patients in need. Table 6-2 depicts the strategies that might be followed for each group of chemically sensitive patients. At this time, patients typically consult clinical ecologists and allergists out of desperation, rather than as a result of referrals. Our considered opinion is that a structured, sensible referral strategy needs to be developed.

Primary care physicians are in the best position to provide knowledgeable referrals for chemically sensitive patients by referring them to the health professional most likely to be of help to the patient. (For a general discussion of the role of the primary care physician in occupational and

TABLE 6-2. Strategies for Primary Care Providers

Group	Primary Referral[a]	Subsequent Referral[a]
Workers	Referral to occupational health physicians or clinics Work histories Industrial hygiene surveys	Clinical ecologists Allergists Detoxification programs where appropriate
Occupants of tight buildings	Adults: For office workers, as above Children: Clinical ecologists or allergists	For office workers, as above
Contaminated communities	With help of State health department, EPA, and/or ATSDR[b] Referral to environmental/ occupational health physicians to take an environmental exposure history	Clinical ecologists Allergists Detoxification progams where appropriate
Individuals		
Pesticides and other toxic substances	As for contaminated communities	As for contaminated communities
Indoor air (domestic)	Clinical ecologists Allergists	

[a] Selected with great care. In our view, this means selecting physicians who take the problem seriously, who do not dismiss these patients' problems as psychiatric without adequate work-up, and who rely upon careful avoidance and judicious reexposure to help determine their patients' sensitivities.

[b] Agency for Toxic Substances and Disease Registry.

environmental medicine, see Institute of Medicine 1988.) Workers exposed to industrial chemicals should be referred to occupational health clinics or occupational physicians. The coupling of industrial hygiene services and a detailed work history help occupational physicians decide what can be done for the chemically exposed patient. In the absence of or in cooperation with an occupational physician, the industrial hygienist may aid primary care physicians in identifying possible illness and relevant exposures. If the problems the worker is experiencing are those of classical toxicity, such as chronic lead poisoning, the occupational physician can help the worker directly. In special cases, such as polybrominated biphenyl (PBB) exposure, some occupational physicians might refer the patient for detoxification therapy to remove the bioaccumulated toxins (Schnare 1986). When the worker is seen to exhibit chemical sensitivity of a nontraditional nature, the occupational physician, if knowledgeable about multiple chemical sensitivity problems, may be able to help the patient. Indeed, many occupational physicians are developing their knowledge in this emerging area. Alternatively, the occupational physician may refer the patient to either a clinical ecologist in whom he has confidence or to an allergist who accepts (recognizes) the problem of multiple chemical sensitivities as real.

Occupants of tight buildings who could be suffering from either classical sensitivity, for example, to molds, or from multiple chemical sensitivities, can also be referred to an occupational health clinic or an occupational physician. The occupational physician may then manage the patient personally or provide the appropriate referral.

For patients that comprise part of a contaminated community, the primary care physician should, ideally, involve the state health department and the EPA or the Agency for Toxic Substances and Disease Registry (ATSDR), which could document exposures and watch for a pattern of illness in that community. (In 1988 the ATSDR [1989, p. 8] awarded a cooperative agreement to support the Association of Occupational and Environmental Health Clinics to expand chemically based information and physicians' educational opportunities relating to toxic substances.) With the assistance of these agencies, the primary care physician can make appropriate referrals to physicians expert in occupational and/or academic environmental medicine. These physicians take an environmental history in much the same manner an occupational physician takes a work history, and this history needs to be coupled both with disease patterns recognized by and with exposure measurements made by the state health and environmental protection departments, EPA, or ATSDR. At that point the occupational or environmental medicine physician can make appropriate referrals to clinical ecologists or allergists in whom he has confidence. Relatively few physicians specialize in environmental medicine. Because environmental medicine and occupational medicine have similar knowledge bases and require many of the same skills, efforts should be directed at developing professionals who span *both* fields in order to serve the chemically sensitive patient.

Finally, for the divergent group of individuals whose illness results from indoor air in the home, pesticide applications, or other chemical exposures, the primary care physician may need to find ways to identify those clinical ecologists and allergists who are able to help the chemically sensitive patient. This group of patients is most challenging because they are diverse and may not fit a particular pattern of illness like the patterns often seen in the workplace, in tight buildings, or as part of a contaminated community. Indeed, some of these patients may not recall a sensitizing event, although they recognize chemical triggers of their symptoms and are polysymptomatic.

The strategies we have outlined for dealing with these four groups of patients need to be carefully developed and refined. The weakest link in affording the patient proper medical care involves raising the consciousness of primary care physicians or those specialists whom the patient might see in a random manner, such as ear, nose, and throat specialists, neurologists, and rheumatologists. However, engaging the primary care physician is the first essential step in sending the patient down a directed pathway of proper referrals. The primary care physician's level of knowledge and concern regarding this problem must be given immediate attention.

The role of the medical specialty societies is central in facilitating the success of these referral strategies. For primary care physicians, including those in family practice, internal medicine, and pediatrics, a clear understanding of the problems of the chemically sensitive patient is requisite. For other specialists, their societies need to address the particular problems of chemical sensitivity that relate to their specialty.

The allergists need to adopt broader perspectives (Kniker 1985), which several allergists seem to be doing. Selner and Staudenmayer (1985b, p. 666) observe:

> It is time for allergy to claim its interest in [the chemical environment] and assume a more active role in the field of toxicology. Allergy is in a position to bring the same disciplined commitment to the principles of scientific investigations to the area of chemical intolerance that has resulted in the remarkable contributions to the field of immunology over the past two decades.

The allergy societies need to commit themselves to a critical but fair appraisal of those techniques and approaches of clinical ecology that may be useful in expanding the practice of allergy beyond its present boundaries. Selner and Staudenmayer (1985a), for example, have stressed the importance of an environmental care unit. Allergists need to be able to take comprehensive work and environmental histories, learn about toxicity and chemical sensitivity, and familiarize themselves with appropriate diagnostic and therapeutic approaches and techniques. Bardana and Montanaro (1989), for example, have suggested that industrial hygiene evaluations of both the workplace and the home "may prove invaluable in identifying chemical sensitivity." The allergy societies should promote the practice of allergy with a broader vision through continuing education efforts and by trying to build on common ground shared with clinical ecology and occupational medicine. Doris Rapp (1985), a board-certified practicing allergist for 18 years and also a clinical ecologist, in response to the position papers of the American Academy of Allergy and Immunology on clinical ecology, cautions:

Try not to wedge the academy in a corner with statements that will haunt allergy in the years to come. If the thinking, leading allergists do not listen, [then] soon, the whole specialty of allergy will be lost. Use your mighty caches of money, and brains to help elucidate our impressive observations and successes. Help us refine what we are doing. Not only will you gain, but the patients, who should be the bottom line of whatever we discuss, will be helped.

The clinical ecologists also need to learn to take better work and environmental histories; to be thorough and not overlook other concomitant medical conditions, for example, hypomagnesemia resulting from a prior partial gastrectomy (Bardana and Montanaro 1989); to engage in continuing educational activities in this rapidly developing area; and to put their work and techniques into a form that would serve as a useful primer for others. The environmental unit is an essential tool for both allergists and clinical ecologists, and their knowledge should be combined in developing new units. The societies whose members practice clinical ecology need to develop rigorous standards for its practices and shun mystical approaches. Bell (1987a) concludes:

Clinical ecology thus needs well-designed, systems-oriented, rigorous interdisciplinary studies. The work must focus on specific diagnostic subgroupings and syndromes as well as on specific immunological and physiological concomitants of adverse reactions. Clinical ecology needs the input of scientists and clinicians from many fields such as public health, occupational medicine, and behavioral medicine, to refine its concepts, treatments, and goals. It otherwise runs the risk of extinction as a fad with several good ideas mingled with too many pernicious and unsubstantiated beliefs.

Finally, clinical ecologists should not simply invoke traditional toxicity as a way of legitimizing the case for avoiding chemical exposures. Mechanisms for multiple chemical sensitivities may be different. Although clinical ecologists may feel pressured to develop a theory of causation, reliance on classical toxicity or allergy, as they are currently understood, may be misplaced.

Recommendations

Having identified the needs of the chemically sensitive person and the community concerned with preventing an increase in the number of chemically affected individuals, we turn to specific recommendations.

Research

States with ATSDR cooperative agreements should establish a registry of chemically sensitive persons with the help of physicians, industrial hygienists, labor organizations, patient-support groups, and others that would be based on physician reports and be as broad as possible to collect data on persons and exposures to be refined and stratified in later analysis. The purpose of the registry is to characterize the nature of the problem and trends over time and to provide a basis for linkage to geographical information system analysis at some time in the future in order to discover sources of exposure.

The federal government should provide funding for a statistically useful questionnaire survey of these persons that stratifies respondents by group, for example, occupationally exposed, occupants of tight buildings, members of contaminated communities, schoolchildren, and the like, and, if possible, by the kind of exposure thought to be responsible for the person's condition, for example, new carpeting, pesticides, and so on. Additionally, states should solicit the financial support of health insurance companies doing business in the state for this effort. State departments of health and ATSDR should analyze the results of the survey in order to identify problem chemicals and affected groups that might serve as the focus for specific field studies.

The federal government should undertake controlled studies of the economic and social effects of indoor air quality on the workforce.

With the assistance of ATSDR, states should undertake field studies of various subgroups of chemically sensitized persons to document their illness. The groups should include occupational groups, contaminated communities, office workers, and children. Studies should involve incidents in which exposures have led to recognized problems, such as certain workplace exposures, toxic waste dumps, contaminated communities, and tight buildings.

The federal agencies (NIH, NIEHS, EPA, and ATSDR) should construct a patient profile of those with chemical sensitivity by evaluating the Environmental Health Center in Dallas. William Rea has agreed in principle to such a study.

The NIH, NIEHS, EPA, NIOSH, and ATSDR should plan a national conference to identify key areas for research into chemical sensitivity that would include allergists, immunologists, clinical ecologists, occupational and environmental physicians, and key governmental researchers.

States should create interagency working groups of state agency professionals to guide the development of state initiatives relevant to the problems of chemical sensitivity.

Information

States should designate one or more professionals to staff a 3-year effort addressing low-level exposures to chemicals. The designated professional (and necessary support staff) should be responsible for preparing written guidelines for the chemically sensitive person designed to provide the affected individual with a clear understanding of the condition and the options for diagnosis, treatment, and compensation. State departments of health should provide a telephone hot line for chemically sensitive individuals in order to guide their inquiries to the appropriate state agencies and offices.

States should request their medical centers to identify, compile, and maintain a list of physicians and clinics interested in handling chemically sensitive patients with consideration, understanding, and relevant medical or other interventions.

State departments of health should prepare educational materials and hold short courses in conjunction with local medical associations to give guidance to primary care physicians in the recognition, diagnosis, treatment, and referral options relevant to chemical sensitivity. Details of possible referral strategies were discussed earlier in this chapter.

The federal agencies should compile and make available emissions data from building materials and consumer products.

States should convene a meeting of those concerned with the design and construction of public and private office buildings and homes to inform them of the problems of indoor air pollution.

Health Care

States should seek funds to enhance the capabilities of existing occupational health clinics to address problems of chemical sensitivity through financial and professional support.

State departments of health should encourage insurance carriers to provide industrial hygiene services for homes and workplaces where multiple chemical sensitivities are suspected. Schools, where problems are indicated, should be investigated by the state.

The federal government, assisted by those experienced in establishing and operating a successful unit, should establish a pilot or demonstration environmental health unit.

The U.S. Department of Education, in consultation with other federal agencies, should evaluate the extent of the problem among schoolchildren and assist states in establishing special classrooms for chemically sensitive children. These special classrooms should be used to study and document the impact of avoidance measures for this subpopulation.

Alternative Employment and Housing

States should educate employers about the chemically sensitive and encourage them to make reasonable accommodations and/or provide alternative worksites within their places of employment and, in some cases, to allow employees to work at home while they improve. States should identify employment options for the chemically sensitive. States should also inform employers and employees of their obligations and rights under federal and state legislation for the handicapped.

Vocational rehabilitation programs, coordinated with programs and activities of state departments of labor and workers' compensation boards, should be established for the chemically sensitive worker.

The state interagency working groups recommended in the Research section ought to be convened to coordinate efforts related to alternative employment and to study housing needs. One option to be studied should be the establishment of halfway houses where newly diagnosed persons or less severely affected persons can recover and receive guidance. Options for the establishment of experimental communities in less polluted environments should also be seriously investigated.

Medical Insurance

The federal government should undertake a study of economic savings that might result from timely and effective medical intervention for chemically sensitive persons.

State departments of health and insurance should use their good offices to express their disapproval of attempts to curb reimbursement for health care for chemically sensitive patients. This effort should be directed towards HCFA, Blue Cross/Blue Shield, and other health insurance carriers. As the problems of the chemically sensitive become better understood, states should do all within their power to facilitate recognition of chemical sensitivity for both health insurance and disability purposes.

Compensation

State departments of health should convene a meeting with the departments of insurance and workers' compensation boards to explain the work-relatedness of chemical sensitivity.

Social and Legal Services

The state interagency working groups recommended in the Research section should study state options for providing access to medically related social and legal services to those whose illness stems from chemical sensitivity.

Regulation of Chemicals

Both state and federal government should consider revising or adding standards to deal with both chemicals that cause initial sensitization and chemicals that trigger sensitivity, that is, low-level exposure to chemicals in the environment, industrial workplace, office, home, and consumer products. Just as no smoking areas are provided in public and private facilities, environmentally acceptable areas could be required. States should work closely with the EPA's Office of Indoor Air Pollution to establish federal policy for chemical sensitivity.

Resolution of Conflicts among Medical Practitioners and Their Societies

Federal and state governments should facilitate dialogue and an easing of antagonisms among allergists, clinical ecologists, and occupational and environmental physicians through educational efforts and through cosponsorship of conferences on chemical sensitivity.

Appendix: Health Effects Associated with Chemicals or Foods

Many, but by no means all, of the articles summarized here were written by clinical ecologists. Indeed, studies by *nonecologists* link rhinitis to laser printers and diesel exhaust; headaches, panic attacks, and kidney problems to solvents; heart arrhythmias to aerosol propellants; balance and memory difficulties to formaldehyde exposure; asthma to carbonless copy paper, perfume, and tobacco smoke; and connective tissue diseases to rocket fuel, vinyl chloride, and hair dye. By presenting this material, we are not affirming an environmental cause for these diseases but hoping to alert the reader to that possibility and the need for evaluating such patients in an environmental unit when more traditional approaches have failed. These references illustrate the range and diversity of health effects that some have associated with chemicals or foods. In some cases, mechanisms may be those of classical allergic sensitivity or toxicity, but for the most part the mechanisms have not yet been elucidated.

Alcoholism. Termed the "ultimate food addiction" by Randolph in the late 1940s (Randolph 1956, 1976c, 1980, pp. 109–116). According to him, people who drink heavily may be sensitive to the food from which the alcoholic beverage is derived. For example, bourbon drinkers may be sensitive to corn and may need to avoid all sources of corn in order to control their cravings (Randolph 1987, pp. 40–47). Individuals may first become aware of a food intolerance when they react adversely to a particular alcoholic beverage, for example, vodka (potatoes), wine (grapes), or bourbon (corn). Alcohol is quickly absorbed so that the individual is more aware of symptoms being associated with a particular alcoholic beverage than with the corresponding food. For example, a person who develops a headache only 3 minutes after drinking bourbon might have a headache 10 to 12 minutes after eating corn sugar or 20 to 25 minutes after cornstarch, and only a scratchy throat 2 to 3 hours after corn oil. The time for symptoms to become manifest thus depends upon the rate of absorption. According to Randolph (1987, p. 184), the majority of alcoholics in this country are addicted to corn; if they manage to abstain from alcohol, they often substitute corn sugar in the form of candy, ice cream, or some other corn-containing food.

Obesity.   According to Philpott (1976), it "characteristically involves addiction to several foods." Insatiable hunger or food cravings may emerge as a withdrawal symptom from certain foods or chemical exposures, making adherence to a weight-reduction diet exceedingly difficult (Randolph 1956). Diets structured around calorie restriction most often fail because foods that the dieter is addicted to and thus craves have not been eliminated. "Suffice it to say, briefly, that obesity and alcoholism are basically similar illnesses, one dealing with addicting foods in their edible form and the other in their potable form" (Randolph 1980, p. 100).

Tobacco Use.   Philpott and associates (1980) reported that 75 percent of schizophrenics he saw in his practice exhibited psychiatric symptoms when smoking cigarettes. Following a 2- to 3-week period of abstinence (deadaptation), 10 percent became psychotic upon reexposure to tobacco smoke. Many physicians recall with displeasure how smoky psychiatric ward lounges were when they rotated through psychiatry as students and recall being taught to allow a patient who seemed to be decompensating the opportunity to smoke a cigarette.

Tobacco belongs to the nightshade food family along with potato, tomato, eggplant, and green pepper. Smokers, who are addicted to tobacco, may have sensitivities to these foods as well; paradoxically, sensitivity may result in either a strong dislike for these foods or a craving for them, that is, addiction (Randolph 1987, p. 253).

Cardiac and Vascular Disease

Rea (1975, 1977, 1981, 1987c), a thoracic surgeon prior to his involvement with clinical ecology, reviews cardiovascular disease from the clinical ecologists' perspective.

Arrhythmias. See the Rea references for cardiac and vascular disease and also Boxer (1976) and Seyal (1986b, 1986d).

Vasculitis. See Cardiac and Vascular Disease.

Thrombophlebitis. See Cardiac and Vascular Disease.

Hypertension. Increased blood pressure, heart rate, and arrhythmias are attributed to the wearing of synthetic clothing versus cotton clothing by Seyal (1986b, 1986c).

Angina and Myocardial Infarctions. Numerous studies outside clinical ecology support the idea that environmental agents may trigger cardiac symptoms. Kalsner and Richards (1984) reported in *Science* that histamine levels are increased in coronary arteries of cardiac patients, suggesting that "an 'allergic' response as occurs in an antigen-antibody type reaction could induce a powerful contraction or spasm of a coronary vessel segment and precipitate a cardiac crisis such as angina or rhythm disruption." Nitroglycerin is widely recognized to be able to provoke angina as well as mitigate it (see Chapter 2). Fluorocarbons in aerosol propellants may precipitate arrhythmias (Speizer et al. 1975; Taylor and Harris 1970). See also the Rea references for cardiac and vascular disease and Seyal (1987/88).

Edema and Fluid-Retention Syndromes. See Cardiac and Vascular Disease.

Eye, Ear, Nose, and Throat Disorders

Ear, nose, and throat (ENT) symptoms secondary to environmental triggers may be a common early warning sign of environmental hyperreactivity, with heightened awareness and intolerance of odors being one of the most common symptoms. Roughly 20 percent of ENT physicians practice allergy themselves and perhaps about one third of these physicians are interested in chemical sensitivity. Some refer their patients with multisystem complaints to clinical ecologists. See Rea (1979a, 1979b).

Eye Disorders.   For conjunctivitis, eczema of the eyelids, blurring of vision, tearing, light sensitivity (photophobia), and other eye problems, see Rapp and Bamberg (1986); Rapp (1978b); Sandberg (1987b); also indices of Randolph and Moss (1980) for individual cases.

Laryngeal Edema.   Using videoendoscopy of the larynx, LaMarte and co-workers (1988) documented laryngeal edema in a patient exposed to the alkylphenol novolac resin used in making carbonless carbon paper. Concomitantly, plasma histamine levels rose sixfold from prechallenge levels. Similarly Selner and Staudenmayer (1985b) showed spasm of the pharyngeal constrictor muscles in a woman exposed to copy machine emissions when challenged in a blinded fashion with sham challenges as controls.

Meniere's Disease.   See Eye, Ear, Nose, and Throat Disorders.

Otitis Media.   Bernstein (1988) reported 2 to 3 times more serum IgE directed against milk, eggs, and wheat among a group of 10 otitis-prone children (six or more episodes in first 2 years of life) compared to 18 controls (less than four episodes in the first 2 years). See also Rea (1979a, 1979b), Pelikan (1987), Shambaugh (1983), and Boris et al. (1985b).

Rhinitis, Frequent Colds, Chronic Nasal Obstruction.   Skoner and associates (1990) describe "laser printer rhinitis" in a 51-year-old man who experienced nasal congestion, skin irritation, headache, and chest and stomach discomfort when a new computer and laser printer were installed at his work station. Blinded challenge confirmed that laser printed paper, which emits various volatile organic compounds, including combustion products from styrene-butadiene toners, caused a three- to four-fold increase in nasal airway resistance as measured by computerized posterior rhinomanometry. See also Rea (1979a, 1979b) and Pelikan (1987).

Salivary Gland Disorders.   See Eye, Ear, Nose, and Throat Disorders.

Sinusitis.   See Eye, Ear, Nose, and Throat Disorders.

Vertigo, Hearing Loss, Tinnitus, Pressure in Ear.   See Rea (1979a, 1979b), Odkvist et al. (1985), and Powers (1976).

Endocrine Disorders

See generally Saifer and Becker (1987).

Thyroid Dysfunction. Gaitan and associates (1985) hypothesize that organic and microbial water pollutants may be responsible for an increased incidence of goiter and autoimmune thyroiditis in certain regions. Polychlorinated biphenyls (PCBs) and polybrominated biphenyls (PBBs) may interfere with thyroid hormone secretion (Bastomsky 1985). Of workers at a plant manufacturing PBBs, 11 percent were hypothyroid and showed increased titers of thyroid antimicrosomal antibodies, perhaps from a PBB-induced autoimmune response (Bahn et al. 1980).

Premenstrual Syndrome. See Rea (1988b), Mabray et al. (1982), and Mabray (1982/1983).

Fatigue

Randolph's (1945, 1947, 1980, pp. 138–146) writings on this subject extending back to the 1940s suggest that fatigue syndrome, an illness currently the subject of great discussion among physicians, might be investigated on this basis (environmental unit, fasting). Indeed, Randolph reported seeing many atypical lymphocytes in the peripheral blood smears of chronic allergic patients, resembling mononucleosis, which has been linked by some to chronic fatigue syndrome (Randolph 1945). Fatigue is reportedly one of the most common manifestations of food and chemical sensitivity and resolves with avoidance of incriminated foods and chemicals. Drowsiness following a meal is said to be a common sign of food sensitivity. Features of chronic fatigue syndrome (Jessop 1990), such as its age of onset; female predominance; polysymptomatic complaints, especially neurological ones; normal examinations and routine lab findings; carbohydrate cravings; recurrent yeast infections; and immunologic abnormalities, such as frequent low titers of autoantibodies and altered cellular immunity, are strikingly similar to the features of multiple chemical sensitivity.

Gastrointestinal Disorders

Certain digestive tract disorders are clearly linked to foods; for example, gluten sensitive enteropathy is associated with wheat consumption.

However, traditional gastroenterologists doubt or remain uncertain about the role of foods in many conditions.

The following papers concern food as triggers of gastrointestinal disorders; however, chemical exposures are also reported (see Randolph's books) to result in increased food intolerance, bloating, heartburn, and other gastrointestinal manifestations.

Oral Manifestations Including Aphthous Ulcers. See Challacombe and Walker-Smith (1987), Ford (1987), and Hindle and Franklin (1986).

Celiac Disease (Gluten-Sensitive Enteropathy). See Mike and Asquith (1987).

Enterocolitis in Infants. See Van Sickle et al. (1985). Lymphocytes from infants with milk or soy intolerance (demonstrated by oral food challenge) had an augmented response to mitogen stimulation when cultured with soy protein or milk protein.

Gastroenteritis. See Trounce and Tanner (1985). Gross and co-workers (1989) describe a physician who was hospitalized four times and underwent biopsies of his esophagus, stomach, small bowel (three times), liver, bone marrow, gums, and skin in an effort to find the cause of his severe abdominal cramps. An elimination diet helped to identify yellow dye #6 as the offending agent. It was confirmed with double-blind challenge.

Inflammatory Bowel Disease. See Shorter (1987).

Chronic Ulcerative Colitis. Food sensitivity was proposed as the principal cause of ulcerative colitis by Rowe in 1942. See Rowe (1949) and McEwen (1987).

Irritable Bowel Syndrome. Jones and Hunter (1987) found that specific foods induced symptoms of irritable bowel syndrome in 14 of 21 patients; double-blind food challenges with six patients confirmed food intolerance. See also Jones (1982).

Gynecological Disorders

See Mabray et al. (1982) and Mabray (1982/1983, 1983).

Dysmenorrhea (Painful Menses). See Gynecological Disorders.

Premenstrual Syndrome (PMS).   See the Mabray references and also Rea (1988b).

Infertility.   See Gynecological Disorders.

Fibrocystic Breast Disease (Breast Tenderness).   Russell (1989) demonstrated that breast pain can be mitigated by eliminating caffeine from the diet. A study published in the *Journal of Allergy and Clinical Immunology* found that the total methyl xanthine content in the diet (including tea, coffee, chocolate, colas, and theophylline, which is used to treat asthma) was predictive of fibrocystic breast disease severity (Hindi-Alexander et al. 1985). Other papers confirm this relationship (Boyle et al. 1984) or dispute it (Levinson and Dunn 1986; Lubin et al. 1985). Jacobson and Liebman (1986) discussed the limitation of case-controlled studies of fibrocystic breast disease; such studies can easily miss an association if not all cases have the same disease or if all individuals are not equally sensitive to methyl xanthines. Interestingly, Jacobson and Liebman felt further case-controlled studies would be futile and suggested instead double-blind controlled challenges to resolve the debate once and for all.

More recently, Russell (1989) counseled 138 women with documented fibrocystic breast disease to reduce their caffeine intake. Of 113 women (81.9 percent) who decreased their caffeine consumption significantly, 69 (61 percent) experienced lessening of breast pain versus 21 percent of women who did not decrease their caffeine intake. See also the Mabray references.

Hematological Abnormalities

Anemia.   See Heiner et al. (1962). IgE is clearly involved in Heiner's syndrome, in which milk consumption results in anemia, poor weight gain, gastrointestinal symptoms, severe recurrent lung disease, and upper respiratory tract symptoms; other concomitant mechanisms play a role in this syndrome.

Thrombocytopenia.   See Caffrey and others (1981).

Neurobehavioral and Psychiatric Manifestations

Randolph (1980) describes the stimulatory and withdrawal effects of environmental incitants (see Chapter 2) and their psychiatric correlates, ranging from hyperactivity (+ +), autism, anxiety, mania, panic attacks, and seizures (+ + + +) at the furthest extreme, to withdrawal levels, including "brain fag," that is, impaired thinking ability (− − −), and severe depression (− − −, − − − −). King (1981) performed double-blind sublingual testing on 30 patients who complained of at least one psychological symptom by using conventional allergy food extracts as well as tobacco smoke extract and was able to provoke cognitive-emotional symptoms more frequently using these incitants than placebo (*p* = 0.001). See also Pearson and Rix (1987), Bell and King (1982), and Bell (1982, 1987a, 1987b).

Affective Disorders (Depression, Mania). See Bell (1987a) and Randolph (1980, pp. 147–155).

Anxiety and Somatoform Disorder. Bell (1987a) cautions: "Psychological diagnoses such as somatization disorder are always diagnoses of exclusion of organic factors. If a double-blind study is inadequately designed, researchers might miss a true biological effect and mistakenly conclude a psychogenic basis for the presenting complaints. In addition, the finding of psychological factors does not rule out biological components to a phenomenon." (See also Chapter 4.)

Sexual Dysfunction. See Randolph (1976f).

Eating Disorders. See Bell (1987a).

Hyperactivity. Using a blinded study design, Kaplan and associates (1989) provided a replacement diet free of food additives and stimulants and low in simple sugars to 24 hyperactive preschool boys. In addition, any foods implicated by parents were avoided, and an attempt was made to reduce exposure to common environmental inhalants. Forty-two percent of the children showed approximately 50 percent improvement in behavior on the diet as well as having less halitosis, night awakenings, and difficulty getting to sleep. The authors stress that had they eliminated and tested only a *single* type of substance, such as sugar or dyes, as in others' studies, 10 percent or fewer of the children would have shown improvement.

See also Egger (1987b) and Rapp and Bamberg (1986).

Schizophrenia. See "Tobacco Use" in this section. Philpott (1976, p. 16) wrote that the schizophrenic patient usually is sensitive to a wide assortment of substances. Foods most likely to provoke reactions included wheat (64 percent), corn (51 percent), and milk (50 percent). Tobacco and coffee also produced symptoms frequently. Avoidance of smoking improved psychosis in some schizophrenic patients, and rechallenge exacerbated their psychotic symptoms. King (1985) reviewed studies of wheat gluten as a factor in schizophrenia and reported that the studies with more adequate statistical power were positive and suggest that wheat gluten may provoke schizophrenic symptoms. See also Bell (1987a).

Panic Disorder.   Panic disorder has been associated with organic solvent exposure (Dager 1987) and caffeine consumption (Boulenger 1984). In one study, 20 patients with panic disorder were exposed to 5.5 percent carbon dioxide–enriched air, a mixture that provokes attacks in most patients with panic disorder (Sanderson 1989). All patients were told that illumination of a light in front of them would signal that they could dial downward the amount of CO_2 they were receiving. In fact, the dials were nonfunctional. For ten of the patients, the light was illuminated the entire time CO_2 was administered; for the other ten, it was not illuminated at all. Patients who believed they had control of the CO_2 experienced fewer and less intense panic disorder symptoms, suggesting that psychological factors (the illusion of control) can influence the biological response to a physical stressor.

Neurological Disorders

The occupational health literature is replete with reports of neurological impairment attributed to various chemicals, many of which were not previously recognized for these effects. Whether certain of these neurological sequelae represent a facet of the multiple chemical sensitivity syndrome or are subtle toxic effects not previously recognized remains to be determined. For example, formaldehyde, which for decades was considered an irritant, has now been linked with protracted impairment of memory, equilibrium, and dexterity in histology technicians (Kilburn 1987). Knowing if those technicians most affected by formaldehyde also experience central nervous system or multisystem effects from other chemical exposures such as perfume and diesel exhaust would be useful.

Headaches of almost any description (tension, migraine, "sinus") are considered by ecologists to be common manifestations of food and chemical intolerance (Randolph 1979). Randolph cautions that "headache diets" most often do not relieve the patient's symptoms either because they fail to exclude certain key foods or because important chemical exposures are not avoided. No single diet works for *all* patients; foods must be tested for each individual. Frequently patients note that a particular food relieves their headache yet are unaware that the same food may also be the cause (Randolph 1980, pp. 123–128).

Migraine. See Monro (1987), Egger (1987a), Egger and co-workers (1983, 1989), and Mansfield and associates (1985). See also "Seizure Disorders."

Seizure Disorders. Egger (1989) found improvement in 40 of 45 children with epilepsy *and* migraine placed on an oligo-antigenic elimination diet; complete control of seizures was achieved with 25 patients; double-blind, placebo-controlled challenges conducted in eight patients provoked seizures. None of 18 patients with epilepsy alone improved. Alternation between seizures (+ + + +) and headache (− −) (see Table 2-2) in some individuals is recognized by neurologists, but the mechanism is not known. Randolph's (1980) description of the levels of addiction provides a possible context for understanding this phenomenon. See also Bell (1987a).

A Swedish study found that 7.7 percent of 104 subjects with focal epilepsy had significant exposure to organic solvents in their jobs, for example, painters (Littorin 1988).

Sleep Disorders. Sleep apnea, hypersomnia, narcolepsy, and restless legs syndrome are discussed in Bell (1987a).

Pulmonary Disorders

Asthma. Bronchospasm in certain workers exposed to toluene di-iso-cyanate and certain other industrial chemicals is undisputed among medical practitioners; however, such responses to tobacco smoke or perfume are often questioned or dismissed as irritant reactions. Shim and Williams (1986), pulmonary specialists, challenged four asthmatics with cologne for 10 minutes; their pulmonary function tests (FEV_1) dropped 18 to 58 percent below baseline. Of 60 asthmatics they surveyed, 57 complained of respiratory symptoms with exposure to common "odors": insecticide (85 percent), household cleaners (78 percent), perfume or cologne (72 percent), cigarette smoke (75 percent), fresh paint (73 percent), auto exhaust fumes (60 percent), and cooking smells (37 percent).

Gerdes and Selner (1980) studied a 35-year-old steroid-dependent asthmatic who complained of worsening bronchospasm after eating corn. Double-blind challenges with D_5NS (intravenous normal saline with 5 percent dextrose, a corn-derived sugar) and plain normal saline showed a reproducible decrement in pulmonary function after dextrose only.

Stankus and associates (1988) studied 21 asthmatics (19 atopic) who complained of cough, shortness of breath, and chest tightness with exposure to cigarette smoke. Seven of 21 experienced significant, reproducible reductions in their ability to perform pulmonary function tests (more than 20 percent decrease in FEV_1) when exposed to cigarette smoke for 2 hours. The gradual declines in FEV_1 that occurred were unlike the usual early or late responses induced by classic allergen inhalation testing, and there was no association with serum IgE antibodies or skin tests to tobacco leaf extract. Accordingly, the authors comment that the mechanism of bronchospasm from cigarette smoke is unclear. Of interest is their finding that the other 14 asthmatics who claimed they were sensitive to cigarette smoke did *not* experience bronchospasm with challenge testing. These individuals might have shown positive challenges if the testing had been done while they were in the deadapted state, that is, after an appropriate interval (such as 4 to 7 days) away from cigarette smoke. Some of these individuals may have avoided smoke for weeks or longer and thus have lost their sensitivity.

Rodriguez de la Vega et al. related asthma in Cuba to exposures to kerosene fuel (Rodriguez de la Vega 1990). Of 286 asthmatic women followed for five years, only 15.5 percent of those who improved clinically had contact with kerosene, while 43.9 percent of those who failed to improve used kerosene as a cooking fuel. In 16 of the women, asthma began soon after they began using kerosene.

A variety of food additives, including sulfites (Bush 1986) and monosodium glutamate (Allen 1987), have been shown in blinded, placebo-controlled challenges to provoke asthma in certain individuals. See also Wraith (1987) and Hoj and co-workers (1981).

Pneumonitis. See Heiner and associates (1962) and also "Anemia."

Renal and Urological Disorders

See Sandberg (1987) and Dickey (1976).

Enuresis (Bedwetting). See Gerrard and Zaleski (1976).

Glomerulopathy. Finn et al. (1980) report increased occupational exposure to hydrocarbons among patients whose renal failure resulted from glomerular nephritis. See also McCrory and associates (1986).

Nephrotic Syndrome.   Sandberg et al. (1977) discuss six cases of severe idiopathic nephrotic syndrome that were related to milk ingestion. See also Sandberg (1987a) and Dickey (1976).

Rheumatological Disorders

See Wojtulewski (1987).

Lupus Erythematosus.   Reidenberg and co-workers (1983) report the case of a laboratory worker exposed to hydrazine who developed a lupuslike syndrome with arthralgias, fatigue, malar (cheek) rash, photosensitivity, antinuclear antibody, and antibodies to native DNA. Symptoms cleared away from work and returned when an in-hospital challenge test with hydrazine was performed. Her lymphocytes, but not those of three normal controls, showed inhibition of mitogen-stimulated IgG synthesis following five daily exposures to hydrazine. Two major drugs, procainamide and hydralazine, which contain hydrazine moieties in their chemical structures, are widely recognized as causing lupuslike diseases. Hydrazine also occurs in a wide variety of natural and synthetic substances (over 30 million pounds of hydrazine are used by industry in the United States each year) such as mushrooms, tobacco smoke, plastics, rubber products, herbicides, pesticides, photographic supplies, textiles, dyes, and drugs. Tartrazine (FD&C yellow #5), which is found in thousands of foods and drugs, can be metabolized to hydrazine compounds and has been linked to one case of a lupuslike syndrome.

Scleroderma.   Scleroderma-like syndromes (scleroderma is a connective tissue disorder that can affect the skin, lung, esophagus, and other tissues) have been linked to a variety of environmental exposures including vinyl chloride, silica dust, organic solvents, epoxy resins, and ingestion of toxic cooking oil in Spain (Black 1988). Specific features of the illnesses resulting from each type of exposure vary somewhat, but overlap is significant. Other exposures that have been related to scleroderma-like illnesses include various drugs, breast augmentation (paraffin and silicone), and use of hair dyes (Fremi-Titulaer 1989). Hair dyes contain aromatic amines that are absorbed through the scalp and metabolized by acetylation in the liver. Individuals who are slow acetylators, that is, those whose enzymes do not break down these amines as readily, may be at greater risk for the disease.

Myalgia and Arthralgia.   According to Randolph (1976d), myalgias, arthralgias, and pain associated with both osteoarthritis and rheumatoid arthritis improve when incriminated food and chemical incitants are avoided.

Rheumatoid Arthritis. In 1976 the American Arthritis Foundation concluded, "No food has anything to do with causing arthritis, and no food is effective in treating or curing it" (Skoldstam 1989). However, some rheumatologists have identified a few patients who seem to benefit from special diets. (See also Randolph 1976d.)

Kroker and associates (1984) and Marshall and associates (1984) describe a multicenter study conducted by clinical ecologists in which 43 patients with rheumatoid arthritis entered an environmental unit and underwent fasting followed by food challenge. Seven parameters of arthritis activity were measured, and all significantly improved during the fast ($p = 0.001$). Following challenge with provoking foods in 27 patients, joint pain and circumference increased, while grip strength decreased ($p = 0.001$).

Panush (1986a, 1986b), a rheumatologist, showed that rheumatoid arthritis improved significantly in 2 of 11 patients on a restricted diet (foods were not individually tested, nor were patients in an environmental unit). In the two patients who improved, symptoms recurred when they deviated from their diet, and double-blind food challenges demonstrated that specific foods exacerbated their symptoms. One wonders if more patients might have improved had foods been tested on an individual basis in a chemically controlled environment, as was done in the clinical ecology study. The clinical ecologists followed a more strict elimination diet (fasting) than did Panush. In addition, chemical exposures were controlled because ecologists' patients were in an environmental unit.

In an interesting animal study, Coombs and Oldham (1981) placed rabbits on cow's milk instead of water for 12 weeks and induced knee joint synovitis, in some cases quite severe. See also Randolph (1976d).

Other Arthritides. Randolph (1980, p. 130) is of the opinion that Reiter's syndrome, ankylosing spondylitis, psoriatic arthritis, and other types of arthritis may also have environmental bases.

Skin Diseases

Atopic Dermatitis (Eczema). That IgE-mediated food sensitivities have a role in some cases of atopic dermatitis is gaining wider acceptance by allergists and dermatologists. Studies have shown that at least one third of patients presenting to allergists or dermatologists with this condition have underlying food allergies (Burks et al. 1988). In addition to provoking skin symptoms, 30 percent of positive food challenges also resulted in gastrointestinal symptoms (nausea, vomiting, abdominal pain, or diarrhea) and 52 percent in respiratory symptoms (wheezing, nasal congestion, or sneezing). In select (referred) patients with eczema, Sampson (1985) found that foods provoked symptoms in about 56 percent of those who underwent double-blind, placebo-controlled food challenges. See also Pike and Atherton (1987).

Dermatitis Herpetiformis.   See Leonard and Fry (1987). That dermatitis herpetiformis is associated with gluten-sensitive enteropathy (celiac disease) and that gluten (for example, from wheat) plays a causal role in both this rash and the enteropathy are widely accepted.

Urticaria.   See Winkelmann (1987). Allergists recognize that a wide variety of foods and additives, including caffeine (Pola et al. 1988), can be potential triggers for urticaria and exercise-induced anaphylaxis. Contact urticaria and airway obstruction in response to carbonless copy paper have been reported (Marks et al. 1984). Delayed pressure urticaria has also been observed to clear during fasting and to recur with food challenge (Davis et al. 1986).

Bibliography

Agency for Toxic Substances and Disease Registry (ATSDR), *Annual Report for FY 1988,* May (1989).

Akiyama, K., et al., "Hapten-modified Basophils: A Model of Human Immediate Hypersensitivity that Can Be Elicited by IgG Antibody," *Journal of Immunology* (1984) 133(6):3286–3290.

Allen, D., et al., "Monosodium L-glutamate-induced Asthma," *Journal of Allergy and Clinical Immunology* (1987) 80(4):530–537.

American Academy of Allergy and Immunology, "Position Statements—Allergen Standardization," *Journal of Allergy and Clinical Immunology* (1980) 66(6):431.

———, "Position Statements—Controversial Techniques," *Journal of Allergy and Clinical Immunology* (1981) 67(5):333–338.

———, "Position Statements—Clinical Ecology," *Journal of Allergy and Clinical Immunology* (1986) 72(8):269–271.

American College of Physicians, "Clinical Ecology," *Annals of Internal Medicine* (1989) 111(2):168–178.

Angyal, A., *Neurosis and Treatment,* Revised Edition (1981), Hanfman, E., et al. (eds.) Unpublished manuscript.

Ashford, N., "New Scientific Evidence and Public Health Imperatives," *Environmental Impact Assessment Review* (1987) 7:203–206.

Ashford, N., et al., "Human Monitoring: Scientific, Legal and Ethical Considerations," *Harvard Environmental Law Review* (1984) 8(2):263–364.

ATSDR. See Agency for Toxic Substances and Disease Registry.

Bahn, A., et al., "Hypothyroidism in Workers Exposed to Polybrominated Biphenyls," *New England Journal of Medicine* (1980) 302(1):31–33.

Bailey, K., and Vanderslice, R., "Volatilization of Drinking Water Contaminants While Showering" (1987). Unpublished manuscript.

Bardana, E., Jr., and Montanaro, A., " 'Chemically Sensitive' Patients: Avoiding the Pitfalls," *Journal of Respiratory Diseases* (1989) 10(1):32–45.

Barrett, K., and Metcalfe, D., "The Mucosal Mast Cell and Its Role in Gastrointestinal Allergic Diseases," *Clinical Reviews in Allergy* (1984) 2:39–53.

Barrow, C., et al., "Sensory Irritation and Incapacitation Evoked by Thermal Decomposition Products of Polymers and Comparisons with Known Sensory Irritants," *Archives of Environmental Health* (1978) 33(2):79–88.

Bascom, R., "Chemical Hypersensitivity Syndrome Study: Options for Action, a Literature Review, and a Needs Assessment," prepared for the State of Maryland Department of Health, February 7, 1989.

Bascom, R., and Willes, S., "Nasal Inhalation Challenge Studies: An Approach to the Study of Health Effects of Indoor Air Pollutants," *Indoor Air '90* Fifth International Conference on Indoor Air Quality and Climate, Toronto, Ontario (1990) 1:295–300.

Bastomsky, C., "Polyhalogenated Aromatic Hydrocarbons and Thyroid Function," *Clinical Ecology* (1985) 3(3):162–163.

Bekesi, J., et al., "Lymphocyte Function of Michigan Dairy Farmers Exposed to Polybrominated Biphenyls," *Science* (1978) 199:1207–1209.

Bell, I., *Clinical Ecology* (1982), Common Knowledge Press, Bolinas, California.

———, "The Biopersonality of Allergies and Environmental Illness." Paper presented at the Eighth Annual International Symposium on Man and His Environment in Health and Disease, Dallas, TX, February 21, 1990.

———, "Effects of Food Allergy on the Central Nervous System." In: Brostoff, J., and Challacombe, S. (eds.) *Food Allergy and Intolerance* (1987a), Bailliere Tindall, Philadelphia, 709–722.

———, "Environmental Illness and Health: The Controversy and Challenge of Clinical Ecology for Mind-Body Health," *Advances* (1987b) 4(3):45–55.

Bell, I., and King, D., "Psychological & Physiological Research Relevant to Clinical Ecology: Overview of Current Literature," *Clinical Ecology* (1982) 1(1):15–25.

Bellinger, D., et al., "Longitudinal Analyses of Prenatal and Postnatal Lead Exposure and Early Cognitive Development," *New England Journal of Medicine* (1987) 316:1037–1043.

Bernstein, J., "New Perspectives on Immunologic Reactivity in Otitis Media with Effusion," *Annals of Otology, Rhinology and Laryngology* (1988) 97(3) Part 2, Supplement 132, 19–23.

Bertschler, J., et al., "Psychological Components of Environmental Illness: Factor Analysis of Changes During Treatment," *Clinical Ecology* (1985) 3(2):85–94.

Besedovsky, H., et al., "Hypothalamic Changes During the Immune Response," *European Journal of Immunology* (1977) 7:323–325.

Black, C., and Welsh, K., "Occupationally and Environmentally Induced Scleroderma-Like Illness: Etiology, Pathogenesis, Diagnosis, and Treatment," *Internal Medicine* (1988) 9(6):135–154.

Bock, S., et al., "Double-Blind, Placebo-Controlled Food Challenge (DBPCFC) as an Office Procedure: A Manual," *Journal of Allergy and Clinical Immunology* (1988) 82(6):986–997.

Bokina, A., et al., "Investigation of the Mechanism of Action of Atmospheric Pollutants on the Central Nervous System and Comparative Evaluation of Methods of Study," *Environmental Health Perspective* (1976) 13:37–42.

Bolla-Wilson, K., et al., "Conditioning of Physical Symptoms after Neurotoxic Exposure," *Journal of Occupational Medicine* (1988) 30(9):684–686.

Boris, M., et al., "Antigen Induced Asthma Attenuated by Neutralization Therapy," *Clinical Ecology* (1985a) 3(2):59–62.

———, "Association of Otitis Media with Exposure to Gas Fuels," *Clinical Ecology* (1985b) 3(4):195–198.

———, "Injection of Low-Dose Antigen Attenuates the Response to Subsequent Bronchoprovocative Challenge," *Otolaryngology—Head and Neck Surgery* (1988) 98(6):539–545.

Boulenger, J., et al., "Increased Sensitivity to Caffeine in Patients with Panic Disorders," *Archives of General Psychiatry* (1984) 41:1067–1071.

Boxer, R., "Cardiac Arrhythmias Due to Foods." In: Dickey, L. (ed.) *Clinical Ecology* (1976), Charles C Thomas, Springfield, IL, 193–200.

Boyle, C., et al., "Caffeine Consumption and Fibrocystic Breast Disease: A Case-Control Epidemiologic Study," *Journal of the National Cancer Institute* (1984) 72(5):1015–1019.

Briere, J., et al., "Summer in the City: Urban Weather Conditions and Psychiatric Emergency-Room Visits," *Journal of Abnormal Psychology* (1983) 92(1):77–80.

Brodsky, C., "Multiple Chemical Sensitivities and Other 'Environmental Illness': A Psychiatrist's View." In: Cullen, M. (ed.) *Workers with Multiple Chemical Sensitivities, Occupational Medicine: State of the Art Reviews* (1987), Hanley & Belfus, Philadelphia, 2(4):695–704.

Brooks, S., et al., "Reactive Airway Dysfunction Syndrome (RADS). Persistent Asthma Syndrome after High Level Irritant Exposures" *Chest* (1985) 88(3):376–384.

Broughton, A., and Thrasher, J., "Antibodies and Altered Cell Mediated Immunity in Formaldehyde Exposed Humans," *Comments in Toxicology* (1988) 2(3):155–174. Gordon and Breach Science Publishers, Great Britain.

Broughton, A., et al., "Immunological Evaluation of Four Arc Welders Exposed to Fumes from Ignited Polyurethane (Isocyanate) Foam: Antibodies and Immune Profiles," *American Journal of Industrial Medicine* (1988) 13:463–472.

―――, "Biological Monitoring of Indoor Air Pollution: A Novel Approach," *Indoor Air '90,* Fifth International Conference on Indoor Air Quality and Climate, Toronto, Ontario (1990) 2:145–150.

Brown, H., et al., "The Role of Skin Absorption as a Route of Exposure for Volatile Organic Compounds (VOCs) in Drinking Water," *American Journal of Public Health* (1984) 74(5):479–484.

Burks, A., et al., "Atopic Dermatitis: Clinical Relevance of Food Hypersensitivity Reactions," *Journal of Pediatrics* (1988) 113(3):447–451.

Bush, R., et al., "A Critical Evaluation of Clinical Trials in Reactions to Sulfites," *Journal of Allergy and Clinical Immunology* (1986) 78(1):191–202.

Butcher, B., et al., "Development and Loss of Toluene Diisocyanate Reactivity: Immunologic, Pharmacologic, and Provocative Challenge Studies," *Journal of Allergy and Clinical Immunology* (1982) 70(4):231–235.

Byers, V., et al., "Association between Clinical Symptoms and Lymphocyte Abnormalities in a Population with Chronic Domestic Exposure to Industrial Solvent–Contaminated Domestic Water Supply and a High Incidence of Leukaemia," *Cancer Immunology Immunotherapy* (1988) 27:77–81.

Caffrey, E., et al., "Thrombocytopenia Caused by Cow's Milk," *Lancet* (August 8, 1981):316.

Calabrese, E., *Pollutants and High Risk Groups: The Biological Basis of Increased Human Susceptibility to Environmental and Occupational Pollutants* (1978), John Wiley & Sons, New York.

Caplin, I., "Report of the Committee on Provocative Food Testing," *Annals of Allergy* (1973) 31:375–381.

Carmichael, P., et al., "Sudden Death in Explosives Workers," *Archives of Environmental Health* (1963) 7:50–65.

Challacombe, S., "Oral Manifestations of Food Allergy and Intolerance." In: Brostoff, J., and Challacombe, S. (eds.) *Food Allergy and Intolerance* (1987), Bailliere Tindall, Philadelphia, 511–520.

Claussen, E., Letter to Earon S. Davis, 7 January (1988).

Cone, J., and Hodgson, M. (eds.) *Problem Buildings: Building Associated Illness and the Sick Building Syndrome, Occupational Medicine: State of the Art Reviews* (1989) 4(4):575–802.

Cone, J., et al., "Patients with Multiple Chemical Sensitivities: Clinical Diagnostic Subsets among an Occupational Health Clinic Population." In: Cullen, M. (ed.) *Workers with Multiple Chemical Sensitivities, Occupational Medicine: State of the Art Reviews* (1987), Hanley & Belfus, Philadelphia, 2(4):721–738.

Connolly, D., "Toxics: Too Risky to Insure? Yes, No, Maybe So," *Toxics Law Reporter* (1988) 3(23):715–723.

Coombs, R., and Oldham, G., "Early Rheumatoid-Like Joint Lesions in Rabbits Drinking Cow's Milk," *International Archives of Allergy and Applied Immunology* (1981) 64:287–292.

Cornfeld, R., and Schlossman, S., "Immunologic Laboratory Tests: A Critique of the Alcolac Decision," *Toxics Law Reporter* (1989) 4(14):381–390.

Corwin, A., "A Chemist Looks at Health and Disease," *Proceedings of the Society for Clinical Ecology,* 12th Advanced Seminar, Key Biscayne, FL (1978).

———, "The Allergy Fallacy: Clinical Consequences," *Clinical Ecology* (1985) 3(4):177–182.

Courpas, M., *Indoor Air Pollution: Cause for Concern?* (1988) Congressional Research Service, Washington, D.C., 88–745ENR.

Crayton, J., "Adverse Reactions to Foods: Relevance to Psychiatric Disorders," *Journal of Allergy and Clinical Immunology* (1986) 78(1):243–250.

Cross, C., et al., "Oxygen Radical and Human Disease," *Annals of Internal Medicine* (1987) 107:526–545.

Cullen, M., "The Worker with Multiple Chemical Sensitivities: An Overview." In: Cullen, M. (ed.) *Workers with Multiple Chemical Sensitivities, Occupational Medicine: State of the Art Reviews* (1987a), Hanley & Belfus, Philadelphia, 2(4):655–662.

———, "Multiple Chemical Sensitivities: Summary and Directions for Future Investigators." In: Cullen, M. (ed.) *Workers with Multiple Chemical Sensitivities, Occupational Medicine: State of the Art Reviews* (1987b), Hanley & Belfus, Philadelphia, 2(4):801–804.

Dager, S., et al., "Panic Disorder Precipitated by Exposure to Organic Solvents in the Work Place," *American Journal of Psychiatry* (1987) 144(8):1056–1058.

Dantzer, R., and Kelley, K., "Stress and Immunity: An Integrated View of Relationships Between the Brain and Immune System," *Life Sciences* (1989) 44:1995–2008.

Daum, S., "Nitroglycerin and Alkyl Nitrates." In: Rom, W. (ed.) *Environmental and Occupational Medicine* (1983), Little, Brown and Co., Boston, 639–648.

Davis, E., Personal communication, March, 28, 1989.

Davis, K., et al., "Possible Role of Diet in Delayed Pressure Urticaria, *Journal of Allergy and Clinical Immunology* (1986) 77(4):566–569.

Descotes, J., *Immunotoxicology of Drugs and Chemicals* (1986), Elsevier, New York.

Dickey, L., "Ecology and Urology." In: Dickey, L. (ed.) *Clinical Ecology* (1976), Charles C Thomas, Springfield, IL, 702–707.

Doane, B., "Clinical Psychiatry and the Physiodynamics of the Limbic System." In: Doane, B., and Livingston, K. (eds.), *The Limbic System: Functional Organization and Clinical Disorders* (1986), Raven Press, New York, 285–315.

Doty, R., et al., "Olfactory Sensitivity, Nasal Resistance, and Autonomic Function in Patients with Multiple Chemical Sensitivities," *Archives of Otolaryngology—Head and Neck Surgery* (1988) 114:1422–1427.

DSM III, *Diagnostic and Statistical Manual of Mental Disorders,* Edition 3, American Psychiatric Association (1980), Washington, DC.

Edgar, R., et al., "Air Pollution Analysis Used in Operating an Environmental Control Unit," *Annals of Allergy* (1979) 42(3):166–173.

Egger, J., "Food Allergy and the Central Nervous System in Childhood." In: Brostoff, J., and Challacombe, S. (eds.) *Food Allergy and Intolerance* (1987a), Bailliere Tindall, Philadelphia, 666–673.

———, "The Hyperkinetic Syndrome." In: Brostoff, J., and Challacombe, S., (eds.) *Food Allergy and Intolerance* (1987b), Bailliere Tindall, Philadelphia, 674–687.

Egger, J., et al., "Oligoantigenic Diet Treatment of Children with Epilepsy and Migraine," *Journal of Pediatrics* (1989) 114(1):51–58.

———, "Is Migraine Food Allergy? A Double-blind Controlled Trial of Oligoantigenic Diet Treatment," *Lancet* (1983) 2:865–869.

Elliott, E., "The Future of Toxic Torts: Of Chemophobia, Risk as a Compensable Injury and Hybrid Compensation Systems," *Houston Law Review* (1988) 25:781–786.

Environmental Protection Agency, Office of Air and Radiation, *Report to Congress on Indoor Air Quality,* August, 1989.

———, "EPA Moves to Reduce Chemical Emissions from Carpets," *Environmental News,* April 18, 1990.

Evans, G., et al., "Psychological Reactions to Air Pollution," *Environmental Research* (1988) 45:1–15.

Fauci, A., "The Revolution in the Approach to Allergic and Immunologic Diseases," *Annals of Allergy* (1985) 55:632–633.

Finn, R., et al., "Hydrocarbon Exposure and Glomerulonephritis," *Clinical Nephrology* (1980) 14(4):173–175.

Finnegan, M., et al., "The Sick Building Syndrome: Prevalence Studies," *British Medical Journal* (1984) 289:1573–1575.

Fiore, M., et al., "Chronic Exposure to Aldicarb-Contaminated Groundwater and Human Immune Function," *Environmental Research* (1986) 41(2):633–645.

Ford, R., and Walker-Smith, J., "Paediatric Gastrointestinal Food-Allergic Disease." In: Brostoff, J., and Challacombe, S. (eds.) *Food Allergy and Intolerance* (1987), Bailliere Tindall, Philadelphia, 570–582.

Foster, S., and Chrostowski, P., *Inhalation Exposures to Volatile Organic Contaminants in the Shower* (1987), presented at the 80th annual meeting of APCA (June 21–26).

Fregly, M., "Comments on Cross-Adaptation," *Environmental Research* (1969) 2:435–441.

Freni-Titulaer, L., et al., "Connective Tissue Disease in Southeastern Georgia: A Case-Control Study of Etiologic Factors," *American Journal of Epidemiology* (1989) 130(2):404–409.

Friedman, R., *Sensitive Populations and Environmental Standards* (1981), The Conservative Foundation, Washington, D.C.

Gaitan, E., et al., "Simple Goiter and Auto-immune Thyroiditis: Environmental and Genetic Factors," *Clinical Ecology* (1985) 3(3):158–161.

Galland, L., "Biochemical Abnormalities in Patients with Multiple Chemical Sensitivities." In: Cullen, M. (ed.) *Workers with Multiple Chemical Sensitivities, Occupational Medicine: State of the Art Reviews* (1987) Hanley & Belfus, Philadelphia, 2(4):755–777.

Gammage, R., and Kaye, S. (eds.) *Indoor Air and Human Health* (1985), Lewis Publishers, Chelsea, MI.

Gerdes, K., and Selner, J., "Bronchospasm Following IV Dextrose," abstract in *Annals of Allergy* (1980) 44:48.

———, *Bronchospasm Following IV Dextrose* (1980), presented at the American College of Allergy, 36th Scientific Congress, January 19–23.

Gerrard, J., and Zaleski, A., "Functional Bladder Capacities in Children with Enuresis and Recurrent Urinary Infections." In: Dickey, L. (ed.) *Clinical Ecology* (1976), Charles C Thomas, Springfield, IL, 224–232.

Gershon, S., and Shaw, F., "Psychiatric Sequelae of Chronic Exposure to Organophosphorus Insecticides," *Lancet* (1961) 1:1371–1374.

Gilman, S., and Winans, S., *Manter and Gatz's Essentials of Clinical Neuroanatomy and Neurophysiology* (1982), F. A. Davis Company, Philadelphia.

Girgis, M., "Biochemical Patterns in Limbic System Circuitry: Biochemical-Electrophysiological Interactions Displayed by Chemitrode Techniques." In: Doane B., and Livingston K. (eds.), *The Limbic System: Functional Organization and Clinical Disorders* (1986), Raven Press, New York, 55–65.

Gliner, J., et al., "Pre-exposure to Low Ozone Concentrations Does Not Diminish the Pulmonary Function Responses to Higher Ozone Concentrations," *American Review of Respiratory Diseases* (1983) 127:51–55.

Good, C., and Dadd, D., *Healthful Houses* (1988), Guaranty Press, Bethesda, Maryland.

Gross, P., et al., "Additive Allergy: Allergic Gastroenteritis Due to Yellow Dye Number Six," *Annals of Internal Medicine* (1989) 111(1):87–88.

Gurka, G., and Rocklin, R., "Immunologic Responses During Allergen-Specific Immunotherapy for Respiratory Allergy," *Annals of Allergy* (1988) 61:239–243.

Hackney, J., et al., "Adaptation to Short-term Respiratory Effects of Ozone in Men Exposed Repeatedly," *Journal of Applied Physiology* (1977a) 43(1):82–85.

————, "Effects of Ozone Exposure in Canadians and Southern Californians, Evidence for Adaptation?" *Archives of Environmental Health* (1977b) 32(3):110–116.

Hafler, D., "In Vivo Activated T Lymphocytes in the Peripheral Blood and Cerebrospinal Fluid of Patients with Multiple Sclerosis," *New England Journal of Medicine* (1985) 312(22):1405–1411.

Hattis, D., et al., "Human Variability in Susceptibility to Toxic Chemicals: A Preliminary Analysis of Pharmacokinetic Data from Normal Volunteers," *Risk Analysis* (1987) 7:415–426.

Heiner, D., et al., "Multiple Precipitins to Cow's Milk in Chronic Respiratory Disease," *American Journal of Diseases in Children* (1962) 103:40–60.

Hendrick, D., and Bird, A., "Alveolitis." In: Brostoff, J., and Challacombe, S. (eds.) *Food Allergy and Intolerance* (1987), Bailliere Tindall, Philadelphia, 498–510.

Hill, D., et al., "A Study of 100 Infants and Young Children with Cow's Milk Allergy," *Clinical Review of Allergy* (1984) 2:125–142.

Hindi-Alexander, M., et al., "Theophylline and Fibrocystic Breast Disease," *Journal of Allergy and Clinical Immunology* (1985) 75(6):709–715.

Hindle, M., and Franklin, C., "Food Allergy or Intolerance in Severe Recurrent Aphthous Ulceration of the Mouth," *British Medical Journal* (1986) 292:1237–1238.

Hirzy, J., Personal communication, April 5, 1989.

Hirzy, J., and Morison, R., "Analysis of Problems Related to Installation of Carpet at EPA Headquarters in 1987–8," Submitted for publication to the *Journal of the American Public Health Association* (1989a).

————, *Carpet/4-Phenylcyclohexane Toxicity: The EPA Headquarters Case*, manuscript presented at the Annual Meeting of the Society for Risk Analysis, October 1989b, San Francisco.

Hoj, L., et al., "A Double-Blind, Controlled Trial of Elemental Diet in Severe, Perennial Asthma," *Allergy* (1981) 36(4):257–262.

Horrobin, D., "The Philosophical Basis for Peer Review and the Suppression of Innovation," *Journal of the American Medical Association* (1990) 263(10):1438–1441.

Horvath, S., et al., "Adaptation to Ozone: Duration of Effect," *American Review of Respiratory Diseases* (1981) 123:496–499.

Howard, J., Executive Administrator, American Academy of Environmental Medicine, letter dated May 15, 1989.

Hunter, D., *The Diseases of Occupations* (1978), Hodder and Stoughton, London.

Husman, K., "Symptoms of Car Painters with Long-term Exposure to a Mixture of Organic Solvents," *Scandinavian Journal of Work, Environment and Health* (1980) 6:19–32.

Immerman, F., and Schaum, J., Final Report of the Nonoccupational Pesticide Exposure Study, U.S. EPA, Research Triangle Park, January 23, 1990.

Institute of Medicine, *Role of the Primary Care Physician in Occupational and Environmental Medicine* (1988), National Academy Press, Washington, D.C.

Isaacson, R., *The Limbic System* (1982), Plenum Press, New York.

Jacobson, M., and Liebman, B., "Caffeine and Benign Breast Disease," *Journal of the American Medical Association* (1986) 255(11):1438–1439.

Jackson, R., et al., "Increased Circulating Ia-Antigen-Bearing T cells in Type I Diabetes Mellitus, *New England Journal of Medicine* (1982) 306(13):785–788.

Jasanoff, S., "Science on the Witness Stand," *Issues in Science and Technology* (1989) 6(1):80–87.

Jessop, C., "The Chronic Fatigue Syndrome," presented at the American Academy of Otolaryngic Allergy Post Graduate Symposium in Allergy and Immunology, Phoenix, Arizona, January, 1990.

Jewett, D., et al., "A Double-Blind Study of Symptom Povocation to Determine Food Sensitivity," *New England Journal of Medicine* (1990) 323(7):429–433.

Johnson, A., and Rea, W., *Review of 200 Cases in the Environmental Control Unit, Dallas,* presented at the Seventh International Symposium on Man and His Environment in Health and Disease, February 25–26, 1989, Dallas.

Jones, V., "Food Intolerance: A Major Factor in the Pathogenesis of Irritable Bowel Syndrome," *Lancet* (1982) 1115–1117.

Jones, V., and Hunter, J., "Irritable Bowel Syndrome and Crohn's Disease." In: Brostoff, J., and Challacombe, S. (eds.) *Food Allergy and Intolerance* (1987), Bailliere Tindall, Philadelphia, 555–569.

Kalsner, S., and Richards, R., "Coronary Arteries of Cardiac Patients Are Hyperreactive and Contain Stores of Amines: A Mechanism for Coronary Vasospasm," *Science* (1984) 223:1435–1437.

Kammuller, M., et al., "Chemical-Induced Autoimmune Reactions and Spanish Toxic Oil Syndrome. Focus on Hydantoins and Related Compounds," *Clinical Toxicology* (1988) 26(3–4):157–174.

Kaplan, B., et al., "Dietary Replacement in Preschool-Aged Hyperactive Boys," *Pediatrics* (1989) 83(1):7–17.

Kare, M., "Direct Pathways to the Brain," *Science* (1968) 163:952–953.

Kerr, F., and Pozuelo, J., "Suppression of Physical Dependence and Induction of Hypersensitivity to Morphine by Stereotopic Hypothalamic Lesions in Addicted Rats," *Mayo Clinic Proceedings* (1971) 46:653–665.

Kilburn, K., "Is the Human Nervous System Most Sensitive to Environmental Toxins?" *Archives of Environmental Health* (1989a) 44(6):343–344.

————, et al., "Neurobehavioral Dysfunction in Firemen Exposed to Polychlorinated Biphenyls (PCBs): Possible Improvement after Detoxification," *Archives of Environmental Health* (1989b) 44(6):345–350.

————, "Formaldehyde Impairs Memory, Equilibrium and Dexterity in Histology Technicians: Effects which Persist for Days After Exposure," *Archives of Environmental Health* (1987) 42(2):117–120.

King, D., "Can Allergic Exposure Provoke Psychological Symptoms? A Double-Blind Test," *Biological Psychiatry* (1981) 16(1):3–19.

————, "Psychological and Behavioral Effects of Food and Chemical Exposure in Sensitive Individuals," *Nutrition and Health* (1984) 3:137–151.

————, "Statistical Power of the Controlled Research on Wheat Gluten and Schizophrenia," *Biological Psychiatry* (1985) 20:785–787.

————, "The Reliability and Validity of Provocative Food Testing: A Critical Review," *Medical Hypotheses* (1988) 25:7–16.

King, W., et al., "Provocation-Neutralization: A Two-Part Study;" Part I. The Intracutaneous Provocative Food Test: A Multi-center Comparison Study," *Otolaryngology—Head and Neck Surgery* (1988a) 99(3):263–271.

————, "Provocation-Neutralization: A Two-Part Study; Part II. Subcutaneous Neutralization Therapy: A Multi-center Study," *Otolaryngology—Head and Neck Surgery* (1988b) 99(3):272–277.

————, "Efficacy of Alternative Tests for Delayed-Cyclic Food Hypersensitivity," *Otolaryngology—Head and Neck Surgery* (1989) 101(3):385–387.

Klerman, G., and Weissman, M., "Increasing Rates of Depression," *Journal of the American Medical Association* (1989) 261(15):2229–2235.

Kline, G., et al., "Ascorbic Acid Therapy for Atopic Dermatitis," presented at the annual meeting of the American Academy of Allergy and Immunology, February 1989, San Antonio, Texas.

Kniker, W., "Deciding the Future for the Practice of Allergy and Immunology," *Annals of Allergy* (1985) 55(2):106–113.

Kreiss, K., "The Epidemiology of Building-Related Complaints and Illness." In: Cone, J., and Hodgson, M. (eds.), *Problem Buildings: Building-associated Illness and the Sick Building Syndrome, Occupational Medicine: State of the Art Reviews* (1989), Hanley & Belfus, Philadelphia 4(4):575–592.

Kroker, G., et al., "Acrylic Denture Intolerance in Multiple Food and Chemical Sensitivity," *Clinical Ecology* (1982) 1(1):48–52.

————, "Fasting & Rheumatoid Arthritis: A Multicenter Study," *Clinical Ecology* (1984) 2(3):137–144.

LaMarte, F., et al., "Acute Systemic Reactions to Carbonless Carbon Paper Associated with Histamine Release," *Journal of the American Medical Association* (1988) 260(2):242–243.

Laseter, J., et al., "Chlorinated Hydrocarbon Pesticides in Environmentally Sensitive Patients, *Clinical Ecology* (1983) 2(1):3–12.

La Via, M., and La Via, D., "Phenol Derivatives Are Immunosuppressive in Mice," *Drug and Chemical Toxicology* (1979) 2(1):167–177.

Lebowitz, M., Personal communication, 5 June 1990.

Lehman, C., "A Double-Blind Study of Sublingual Provocative Food Testing: A Study of Its Efficacy," *Annals of Allergy* (1980) 45:144.

Leonard J., and Fry, L., "Dermatitis Herpetiformis." In: Brostoff, J., and Challacombe, S. (eds.) *Food Allergy and Intolerance* (1987) Bailliere Tindall, Philadelphia, 618–631.

Levin, A., Personal communication, July 14, 1989.

Levin, A., and Byers, V., "Environmental Illness: A Disorder of Immune Regulation." In: Cullen, M. (ed.) *Workers with Multiple Chemical Sensitivities* (1987), Hanley & Belfus, Philadelphia, 2(4):669–682.

Levine, S., and Reinhardt, J., "Biochemical Pathology Initiated by Free Radicals, Oxidant Chemicals, and Therapeutic Drugs in the Etiology of Chemical Hypersensitivity Disease," *Orthomolecular Psychiatry* (1983) 12:166–183.

Levinson, W., and Dunn, P., "Nonassociation of Caffeine and Fibrocystic Breast Disease," *Archives of Internal Medicine* (1986) 146(9):1773–1775.

Lipowski, Z., "Psychiatry: Mindless or Brainless, Both or Neither?" *Canadian Journal of Psychiatry* (1988) 34:249–254.

Little, C., "Mediators in Food Allergy." In: Brostoff, J., and Challacombe, S. (eds.) *Food Allergy and Intolerance* (1987), Bailliere Tindall, Philadelphia, 771–780.

Littorin, M., et al., "Focal Epilepsy and Exposure to Organic Solvents: A Case-Referent Study," *Journal of Occupational Medicine* (1988) 30 (10):805–808.

Lockey, R., "Fatalities from Immunotherapy and Skin Testing," *Journal of Allergy and Clinical Immunology* (1987) 79(4):660–677.

Louis, T., et al., "Findings for Public Health from Meta-Analysis," *Annual Review of Public Health* (1985) 6:1–20.

Lubin, F., et al., "A Case-Control Study of Caffeine and Methylxanthines in Benign Breast Disease," *Journal of the American Medical Association* (1985) 253(16):2388–2392.

Mabray, C., "Obstetrics and Gynecology and Clinical Ecology, Part I," *Clinical Ecology* (1982/1983) 1(2):103–114.

———, "Obstetrics and Gynecology and Clinical Ecology, II," *Clinical Ecology* (1983) 1(3, 4):155–163.

Mabray, C., et al., "Treatment of Common Gynecologic-Endocrinologic Symptoms by Allergy Management Procedures," *Obstetrics and Gynecology* (1982) 59(5):560–564.

McCrory, W., et al., "Immune Complex Glomerulopathy in a Child with Food Hypersensitivity," *Kidney International* (1986) 30(4):592–598.

McGovern, J., et al., "Food and Chemical Sensitivity: Clinical and Immunologic Correlates," *Archives of Otolaryngology* (1983) 109:292–297.

———, "The Role of Naturally Occurring Haptens in Allergy," *Annals of Allergy* (1981–82 Supplement) 47:123.

McEwen,L., "A Double-Blind Controlled Trial of Enzyme Potential Hyposensitization for the Treatment of Ulcerative Colitis," *Clinical Ecology* (1987) 5(2):47–51.

MacLean, P., "The Brain in Relation to Empathy and Medical Education," *Journal of Nervous and Mental Disease* (1967) 144(5):374–382.

———, "A Triune Concept of the Brain and Behavior," In: Boag, T., and Campbell, D., *The Hincks Memorial Lectures* (1973), University of Toronto Press, Toronto, Ontario, 6–66.

———, "Culminating Developments in the Evolution of the Limbic System: The Thalamocingulate Division." In: Doane, B., and Livingston, K. (eds.), *Organization and Clinical Disorders* (1986), Raven Press, New York, 1–28.

McLellan, R., "Biological Interventions in the Treatment of Patients with Multiple Chemical Sensitivities." In Cullen, M. (ed.) *Workers with Multiple Chemical Sensitivities, Occupational Medicine: State of the Art Reviews* (1987), Hanley & Belfus, Philadelphia, 2(4):755–777.

MacQueen, G., et al., "Pavlovian Conditioning of Rat Mucosal Mast Cells to Secrete Rat Mast Cell Protease II," *Science* (1989) 243:83–85.

Mage, D., and Gammage, R., "Evaluation of Changes in Indoor Air Quality Occurring over the Past Several Decades." In: Gammage, R., and Kaye, S. (eds.) *Indoor Air and Human Health* (1985), Lewis Publishers, Chelsea, MI, 5–36.

Maller, O., et al., "Movement of Glucose and Sodium Chloride from the Oropharyngeal Cavity to the Brain," *Nature* (1967) 213(2):713–714.

Mansfield, L., et al., "Food Allergy and Adult Migraine: Double Blind and Mediator Confirmation of an Allergic Etiology," *Annals of Allergy* (1985) 55(2):126–129.

Marks, J., et al., "Contact Urticaria and Airway Obstruction from Carbonless Copy Paper," *Journal of the American Medical Association* (1984) 252(8):1038–1040.

Marshall, R., et al., "Food Challenge Effects on Fasted Rheumatoid Arthritis Patients: A Multicenter Study," *Clinical Ecology* (1984) 2(4):181–190.

Maryland State Department of Education, *Indoor Air Quality: Maryland Public Schools* (1987).

Massachusetts, Commonwealth of, *Indoor Air Pollution in Massachusetts,* April 1, 1989.

Meggs, W., Personal communication (1989a).

——— Letter submitted to the editor, *Journal of Occupational Medicine* (1989b).

Metcalfe, D., "Summary and Recommendations," *Journal of Allergy and Clinical Immunology* (1986) 78(1):250–252.

———, quoted in "Pavlov's Rats," *Discover,* May 1989.

Metz, S., "Anti-inflammatory Agents as Inhibitors of Prostaglandin Synthesis in Man," *Medical Clinics of North America* (1981) 65(4):713–53.

Mike, N., and Asquith, P., "Gluten Toxicity in Coeliac Disease and Its Role in Other Gastrointestinal Disorders." In: Brostoff, J., and Challacombe, S. (eds.) *Food Allergy and Intolerance* (1987), Bailliere Tindall, Philadelphia, 521–548.

Miller, C., *Mass Psychogenic Illness or Chemically Induced Hypersusceptibility?* presented at the H.E.W. Symposium on the Diagnosis and Amelioration of Mass Psychogenic Illness, Chicago, May 30–June 1, 1979.

Miller, J., *Food Allergy: Provocative Testing and Injection Therapy* (1972), Charles C Thomas, Springfield, IL.

———, "A Double-Blind Study of Food Extract Injection Therapy: A Preliminary Report," *Annals of Allergy* (1977) 38:185–191.

Molhave, L., "Indoor Air Pollution Due to Organic Gases and Vapors of Solvents in Building Materials," *Environmental International,* Pergamon Press, Elmhurst, NY (1982) 8:117–127.

———, "Dose-Response Relation of Volatile Organic Compounds in the Sick Building Syndrome," *Clinical Ecology* (1986/1987) IV(2):52–56.

Molhave, L., et al., "Human Reactions to Low Concentrations of Volatile Organic Compounds," *Environmental International* (1986) 12:167–175.

Monro, J., "Food-Induced Migraine." In: Brostoff, J., and Challacombe, S. (eds.) *Food Allergy and Intolerance* (1987), Bailliere Tindall, Philadelphia, 632–665.

Monroe, R., "Episodic Behavioral Disorders and Limbic Ictus." In: Doane, K., and Livingston, K. (eds.), *The Limbic System: Functional Organization and Clinical Disorders* (1986), Raven Press, New York, 251–266.

Morey, P., and Shattuck, D., "Role of Ventilation in the Causation of Building-associated Illness," *Problem Buildings: Building-associated Illness and the Sick Building Syndrome, Occupational Medicine: State of the Art Reviews* (1989), Hanley & Belfus, Philadelphia, 4(4):625–642.

Morris, C., and Cabral, J. (eds.), "Reduction of the Human Body Burdens of Hexachlorobenzene and Polychlorinated Biphenyls." In: *Hexachlorobenzene: Proceedings of an International Symposium* (1986), International Agency for Research on Cancer Scientific Publications, Lyon, France, 597–603.

Morrow, L., et al., "PET and Neurobehavioral Evidence of Tetrabromoethane Encephalopathy," *Journal of Neuropsychiatry and Clinical Neurosciences* (1990, forthcoming).

Muranaka, M., et al., "Adjuvant Activity of Diesel-Exhaust Particulates for the Production of IgE Antibody in Mice," *Journal of Allergy and Clinical Immunology* (1986) 77(4):616–623.

Mustafa, M., and Tierney, D., "Biochemical and Metabolic Changes in the Lung with Oxygen, Ozone and Nitrogen Dioxide Toxicity," *American Review of Respiratory Diseases* (1978) 118:1061–1090.

Namba, T., et al., "Poisoning Due to Organophosphate Insecticides," *American Journal of Medicine* (1971) 50:475–492.

Nasr, S., et al., "Concordance of Atopic and Affective Disorders," *Journal of Affective Disorders* (1981) 3:291–296.

National Federation of Federal Employees, Local 2050, press release, December 5, 1989.

National Foundation for the Chemically Hypersensitive, *Cheers* (1989) 1:6, Wrightsville Beach, NC.

National Research Council, *Toxicity Testing, Strategies to Determine Needs and Priorities* (1984), National Academy Press, Washington, D.C.

National Research Council, Board of Environmental Studies and Toxicology, *Workshop on Health Risks from Exposure to Common Indoor Household Products in Allergic or Chemically Diseased Persons,* July 1, 1987.

Nelson, N., "Perspectives on Diesel Emissions Health Research." In: Lewtas, J. (ed.) *Toxicological Effect of Emissions from Diesel Engines* (1982), Elsevier Biomedical, New York, 371–375.

Nero, A., "Controlling Indoor Air Pollution," *Scientific American* (1988) 258(5):42–48.

O'Banion, D., *Ecological and Nutritional Treatment of Health Disorders* (1981), Charles C Thomas, Springfield, IL.

Odell, R., *Environmental Awakening* (1980), Ballinger, Cambridge, MA.

Odkvist, L., et al., "Solvent-induced Central Nervous System Disturbances Appearing in Hearing and Vestibulo-Oculomotor Tests," *Clinical Ecology* (1985) 3(3):149–153.

Olson, L., et al., "Aldicarb Immunomodulation in Mice: An Inverse Dose-Response to Parts Per Billion Levels in Drinking Water," *Archives of Environmental Contamination and Toxicology* (1987) 16(4):433–439.

Otto, D., et al., "Neurobehavioral and Sensory Irritant Effects of Controlled Exposure to a Complex Mixture of Volatile Organic Compounds," *Neurotoxicology and Teratology* (1990). In press.

Ozonoff, D., Personal communication, March 24, 1989.

Ozonoff, D., et al. "Health Problems Reported by Residents of a Neighborhood Contaminated by a Hazardous Waste Facility," *American Journal of Industrial Medicine* (1987) 11:581–597.

Pan, Y., et al., "Aliphatic Hydrocarbon Solvents in Chemically Sensitive Patients," *Clinical Ecology* (1987–1988) 5(2):126–131.

Panush, R., "Delayed Reactions to Foods. Food Allergy and Rheumatic Disease," *Annals of Allergy* (1986) 56:500–503.

Panush, R., et al., "Food-induced (Allergic) Arthritis: Inflammatory Arthritis Exacerbated by Milk," *Arthritis and Rheumatism* (1986) 29(2):220–226.

Patterson, R., et al., "IgG Antibody Against Formaldehyde Human Serum Proteins: A Comparison with Other IgG Antibodies Against Inhalant Proteins and Reactive Chemicals," *Journal of Allergy and Clinical Immunology* (1989) 84(3):359–366.

Payan, D., "Substance P: A Modulator of Neuroendocrine-Immune Function," *Hospital Practice* (Feb. 15, 1989); 24(2):67–80.

Payan, D., et al., "Neuroimmunology," *Advances in Immunology* (1986) 39:299–323.

Pearson, D., and Rix, K., "Psychological Effects of Food Allergy." In: Brostoff, J., and Challacombe, S. (eds.) *Food Allergy and Intolerance* (1987), Bailliere Tindall, Philadelphia, 688–708.

Pelikan, Z., "Rhinitis and Secretory Otitis Media; A Possible Role of Food Allergy." In: Brostoff, J., and Challacombe, S. (eds.) *Food Allergy and Intolerance* (1987), Bailliere Tindall, Philadelphia, 467–485.

Philpott, W., "Allergy and Ecology in Orthomolecular Psychiatry." In: Dickey, L. (ed.) *Clinical Ecology* (1976), Charles C Thomas, Springfield, IL, 729–737.

Philpott, W., et al., "Four-day Rotation of Foods According to Families." In: Dickey, L. (ed.) *Clinical Ecology* (1976), Charles C Thomas, Springfield, IL, 472–486.

———, *Brain Allergies: The Psycho-Nutrient Connection* (1980), Keats Publishing, New Canaan, CT.

Pierson, T. K., et al. "Risk Characterization Framework for Noncancer Endpoints." Proceedings of a Conference on Methodology for Assessing Health Risks from Complex Mixtures in Indoor Air, Arlington, Virginia, April 16–19, 1990.

Pike, M., and Atherton, D., "Atopic Eczema." In: Brostoff, J., and Challacombe, S. (eds.) *Food Allergy and Intolerance* (1987), Bailliere Tindall, Philadelphia, 583–601.

Pola, J., et al., "Urticaria Caused by Caffeine," *Annals of Allergy* (1988) 60(3):207–208.

Powers, "Metabolic and Allergic Aspects of Inner Ear Dysfunction." In: Dickey, L. (ed.) *Clinical Ecology* (1976), Charles C Thomas, Springfield, IL, 637–644.

Randolph, T., "Fatigue and Weakness of Allergic Origin (Allergic Toxemia) to Be Differentiated from Nervous Fatigue or Neurasthenia," *Annals of Allergy* (1945) 3:418–430.

——, "Allergy as a Causative Factor of Fatigue, Irritability, and Behavior Problems of Children," *Journal of Pediatrics* (1947) 31(1):560–572.

——, "Allergic Type Reactions to Industrial Solvents and Liquid Fuels," abstract in *Journal of Laboratory and Clinical Medicine* (1954a) 44(6):910–911.

——, "Allergic Type Reactions to Mosquito Abatement Fogs and Mists," abstract in *Journal of Laboratory and Clinical Medicine* (1954b) 44(6):911–912.

——, "Allergic Type Reactions to Motor Exhaust," abstract in *Journal of Laboratory and Clinical Medicine* (1954c) 44(6):912.

——, "Allergic Type Reactions to Indoor Utility Gas and Oil Fumes," abstract in *Journal of Laboratory and Clinical Medicine* (1954d) 44(6):913.

——, "Allergic Type Reactions to Chemical Additives of Foods and Drugs," abstract in *Journal of Laboratory and Clinical Medicine* (1954e) 44(6):913–914.

——, "Allergic Type Reactions to Synthetic Drugs and Cosmetics," abstract in *Journal of Laboratory and Clinical Medicine* (1954f) 44(6):914.

——, "Depressions Caused by Home Exposures to Gas and Combustion Products of Gas, Oil, and Coal," abstract in *Journal of Laboratory and Clinical Medicine* (1955) 46(6):942.

——, "The Descriptive Features of Food Addiction," *Quarterly Journal of Studies on Alcohol* (1956) 17:198–224.

——, "A Third Dimension of the Medical Investigation," *Clinical Physiology* (1960) 2(1):42–47.

——, *Human Ecology and Susceptibility to the Chemical Environment* (1962), Charles C Thomas, Springfield, IL.

——, "Ecologic Orientation in Medicine: Comprehensive Environmental Control in Diagnosis and Therapy," *Annals of Allergy* (1965) 23:7–22.

——, "Adaptation to Specific Environmental Exposures Enhanced by Individual Susceptibility." In: Dickey, L. (ed.) *Clinical Ecology* (1976a), Charles C Thomas, Springfield, IL, 46–66.

——, "Stimulatory and Withdrawal Levels of Manifestations." In: Dickey, L. (ed.) *Clinical Ecology* (1976b), Charles C Thomas, Springfield, IL, 169–170.

———, "Ecologically Oriented Rheumatoid Arthritis." In: Dickey, L. (ed.) *Clinical Ecology* (1976c), Charles C Thomas, Springfield, IL, 201–212.

———, "Ecologically Oriented Myalgia and Related Musculoskeletal Painful Syndromes." In: Dickey, L. (ed.) *Clinical Ecology* (1976d), Charles C Thomas, Springfield, IL, 213–223.

———, "The Role of Specific Alcoholic Beverages." In: Dickey, L. (ed.) *Clinical Ecology* (1976e), Charles C Thomas, Springfield, IL, 321–333.

———, "The Enzymatic, Acid, Hypoxia, Endocrine Concept of Allergic Inflammation." In: Dickey, L. (ed.) *Clinical Ecology* (1976f), Charles C Thomas, Springfield, IL, 577–596.

———, *Environmental Medicine: Beginnings and Bibliographies of Clinical Ecology* (1987) Clinical Ecology Publications, Fort Collins, CO.

Randolph, T., and Moss, R., *An Alternative Approach to Allergies* (1980), Lippincott & Crowell, New York.

Rapp, D., "Double-Blind Confirmation and Treatment of Milk Sensitivity," *Medical Journal of Australia* (1978a) 1:571–572.

———, "Weeping Eyes in Wheat Allergy," *Transactions of the American Society of Ophthalmologic and Otolaryngic Allergy* (1978b) 18:149–150.

———, "Comments on the Position Paper on Clinical Ecology by the American Academy of Allergy and Immunology" (1985). In: Randolph, T., *Environmental Medicine: Beginnings and Bibliographies of Clinical Ecology* (1987), Clinical Ecology Publications, Fort Collins, CO, 301–307.

Rapp, D., and Bamberg, D., *A Guide for Caring Teachers and Parents; The Impossible Child—In School—At Home* (1986), Practical Allergy Research Foundation, Buffalo, NY.

Rea, W., "Environmentally Triggered Small Vessel Vasculitis," *Annals of Allergy* (1977) 38:245–51.

———, "The Environmental Aspects of Ear, Nose, and Throat Disease: Part I," *Journal of Clinical Ecology, Oto-Rhino-Laryngology & Allergy Digest* (1979a) 41(7):41–56.

———, "The Environmental Aspects of Ear, Nose, and Throat Disease: Part II," *Journal of Clinical Ecology, Oto-Rhino-Laryngology & Allergy Digest* (1979b) 41 (8/9):41–54.

———, "Review of Cardiovascular Disease in Allergy." In: Frazier, C. (ed.) *Bi-Annual Review of Allergy 1979–1980* (1981), Medical Examination Publishing Co., Garden City, NY, 282–347.

———, *Outpatient Information Manual* (1984a) (1988 revision), Environmental Health Center, Dallas.

———, *Clinical Ecology: A Role in Diagnosing Environmental Illness,* presented at the New England Occupational Medicine Association Conference, December 3–4, 1987, Boston.

———, "Chemical Hypersensitivity and the Allergic Response," *Ear, Nose and Throat Journal* (1988a) 67(1):50–56.

———, "Inter-relationships between the Environment and Premenstrual Syndrome." In: Brush, M., and Goudsmit, E. (eds.) *Functional Disorders of the Menstrual Cycle* (1988b) John Wiley & Sons, New York, 135–157.

———, Letter to American College of Physicians, July 14, 1988c.

———, Personal communication, March 10, 1989.

Rea, W., and Brown, O. "Mechanisms of Environmental Vascular Triggering," *Clinical Ecology* (1985) 3(3):122–128.

———, "Cardiovascular Disease in Response to Chemicals and Foods." In: Brostoff, J., and Challacombe, S. (eds.) *Food Allergy and Intolerance* (1987c), Bailliere Tindall, Philadelphia, 737–754.

Rea, W., et al., "Environmentally Triggered Large-Vessel Vasculitis." In: Johnson, J., and Spencer, J. (eds.) *Allergy and Medical Treatment* (1975), Symposia Specialists, Chicago, 185–198.

———, "Elimination of Oral Food Challenge Reaction by Injection of Food Extracts," *Archives of Otolaryngology* (1984b) 110(4):248–252.

———, "T&B Lymphocyte Parameters Measured in Chemically Sensitive Patients and Controls," *Clinical Ecology* (1986a) 4(1):11–14.

———, "Magnesium Deficiency in Patients with Chemical Sensitivity," *Clinical Ecology* (1986b) 4(1):17–20.

———, "Toxic Volatile Organic Hydrocarbons in Chemically Sensitive Patients," *Clinical Ecology* (1987) 5(2):70–74.

Reidenberg, M., et al., "Lupus Erythematosus-like Disease Due to Hydrazine," *American Journal of Medicine* (1983) 75:363–370.

Reynolds, R., and Natta, C., "Depressed Plasma Pyridoxal Phosphate Concentrations in Adult Asthmatics," *American Journal of Clinical Nutrition* (1985) 41:684–688.

Riedel, F., et al., "Effects of SO_2 Exposure on Allergic Sensitization in the Guinea Pig," *Journal of Allergy and Clinical Immunology* (1988) 82(4):527–534.

Riihimaki, V., and Savolainen, K., "Human Exposure to *m*-Xylene. Kinetics and Acute Effects on the Central Nervous System." *Annals of Occupational Hygiene* (1980) 23:411–432.

Rinkel, H., "Food Allergy: The Role of Food Allergy in Internal Medicine," *Annals of Allergy* (1944) 2:115–124.

Rinkel, H., et al., *Food Allergy* (1951) Charles C Thomas, Springfield, IL.

Rinsky, R. A., et al., "Benzene and Leukemia: An Epidemiologic Risk Assessment," *New England Journal of Medicine* (1987) 316:1044–1050.

Robertson, A., et al., "Comparison of Health Problems Related to Work and Environmental Measurements in Two Office Buildings with Different Ventilation Systems," *British Medical Journal* (1985) 291(6492):373–376.

Rodriguez de la Vega, A., et al., "Kerosene-induced Asthma," *Annals of Allergy* (1990) 64(4):362–363.

Roehm, D., "Effects of a Program of Sauna Baths and Megavitamins on Adipose DDE and PCBs and on Clearing of Symptoms of Agent Orange (Dioxin) Toxicity," *Clinical Research* (1983) 32(2):243a.

Rogers, S., "A Practical Approach to the Person with Suspected Indoor Air Quality Poblems," *Indoor Air '90,* Fifth International Conference on Indoor Air Quality and Climate, Toronto, Ontario (1990) 5:345–349.

Root, D., and Lionelli, G., "Excretion of a Lipophilic Toxicant Through the Sebaceous Glands: A Case Report," *J. Toxicol. Cutaneous and Ocular Toxicology* (1987) 6(1):13–17.

Rosenberg, C., *The Cholera Years* (1962), University of Chicago Press, Chicago, 199–200.

Rosenstock, L., "Hospital-based, Academically-Affiliated Occupational Medicine Clinics," *American Journal of Industrial Medicine* (1984) 6:155–158.

Rotton, J., and Frey, J., "Air Pollution, Weather, and Violent Crimes: Concomitant Time-Series Analysis of Archival Data," *Journal of Personality and Social Psychology* (1985) 49(5):1207–1220.

Rousseau, D., et al., *Your Home, Your Health and Well-Being* (1988). Hartley and Marks, Vancouver, British Columbia.

Rowe, A., "Chronic Ulcerative Colitis—An Allergic Disease," *Annals of Allergy* (1949) 7(6):727–819.

Russell, L., "Caffeine Restriction as Initial Treatment for Breast Pain," *Nurse Practicioner* (1989) 14(2):36–40.

Ryan, C., et al., "Cacosmia and Neurobehavioral Dysfunction Associated with Occupational Exposure to Mixtures of Organic Solvents," *American Journal of Psychiatry* (1988) 145(11):1442–1445.

Saifer, P., and Becker, N., "Allergy and Autoimmune Endocrinopathy: APICH Syndrome." In: Brostoff, J., and Challacombe, S. (eds.) *Food Allergy and Intolerance* (1987), Bailliere Tindall, Philadelphia, 781–796.

Salvaggio, J., "Allergy and Clinical Immunology—2001," *Journal of Allergy and Clinical Immunology* (1986) 78(2):253–268.

Salvaggio, J., and Aukrust, L., "Mold-induced Asthma," *Journal of Allergy and Clinical Immunology* (1981) 68(5):327–346.

Sampson, H., "Food Hypersensitivity and Atopic Dermatitis: Evaluation of 113 Patients," *Journal of Pediatrics* (1985) 107(5):669–675.

Sandberg, D., "Food Sensitivity: The Kidney and Bladder." In: Brostoff, J., and Challacombe, S. (eds.) *Food Allergy and Intolerance* (1987a), Bailliere Tindall, Philadelphia, 755–767.

———, "Food Sensitivity: The Eye." In: Brostoff, J., and Challacombe, S. (eds.) *Food Allergy and Intolerance* (1987b), Bailliere Tindall, Philadelphia, 768–770.

Sandberg, D., et al., "Severe Steroid Responsive Nephrosis Associated with Hypersensitivity," *Lancet* (1977) 1(8008):388–391.

Sanderson, W., et al., "The Influence of an Illusion of Control on Panic Attacks Induced via Inhalation of 5.5 percent Carbon Dioxide-Enriched Air," *Archives of General Psychiatry* (1989) 46:157–162.

Scadding, G., and Brostoff, J., "Low Dose Sublingual Therapy in Patients with Allergic Rhinitis Due to House Dust Mite," *Clinical Allergy* (1986) 16:483–491.

Scadding, L., et al., "Poor Sulphoxidation Ability in Patients with Food Sensitivity," *British Medical Journal* (1988) 297(6641):105–107.

Schnare, D., and Robinson, P., "Reduction of the Human Body Burdens of Hexachlorobenzene and Polychlorinated Biphenyls," International Agency for Research on Cancer, Scientific Publications (1986) 77:597–603.

Schnare, D., et al., "Evaluation of a Detoxification Regimen for Fat Stored Xenobiotics," *Medical Hypotheses* (1982) 9(3):265–282.

————, "Body Burden Reductions of PCBs, PBBs and Chlorinated Pesticides in Human Subjects," *Ambio* (1984) 13(5–6):378–380.

Schottenfeld, R., "Workers with Multiple Chemical Sensitivities: A Psychiatric Approach to Diagnosis and Treatment." In: Cullen, M. (ed.) *Workers with Multiple Chemical Sensitivities* (1987), Hanley & Belfus, Philadelphia, 2(4):739–754.

Selner, J., "Chemical Sensitivity." In: *Current Therapy in Allergy, Immunology and Rheumatology* (1988), B.C. Decker, Philadelphia, 48–52.

Selner, J., and Staudenmayer, H., "The Relationship of the Environment and Food to Allergic and Psychiatric Illness." In: Young, S., and Rubin, J. (eds.), *Psychobiology of Allergic Disorders* (1985a), Praeger, New York, 102–146.

————, "The Practical Approach to the Evaluation of Suspected Environmental Exposures: Chemical Intolerance," *Annals of Allergy* (1985b) 55(5):665–673.

Selye, H., "The General Adaptation Syndrome and the Diseases of Adaptation," *Journal of Allergy* (1946) 17:231–247, 289–323, 358–398.

————, *The Stress of My Life* (1977), McClelland and Stewart, Toronto.

Seyal, A., et al., "Psychosomatic Cardiovascular Disorders: An Elusive Relationship to the Type of Clothing Worn," *Clinical Ecology* (1986a) 4(1):26–30.

————, "Systolic Blood Pressure, Heart Rate and Premature Ventricular Contractions in a Population Sample: Relationship to Cotton and Synthetic Clothing," *Clinical Ecology* (1986b) 4(2):69–74.

————, "A Relationship of Quality of Garments to Blood Pressure in Young School Children," *Clinical Ecology* (1986c) 4(3):115–119.

————, "Premature Ventricular Contractions: The Relationship of Synthetic vs. Natural Fabrics Worn Next to the Skin," *Clinical Ecology* (1986d) 4(4):149–154.

————, "The Influence of Cotton and Synthetic Fabrics on Nocturnal Angina," *Clinical Ecology* (1987/88) 5(3):121–125.

Shakman, R., "Nutritional Influences on the Toxicity of Environmental Pollutants," *Archives of Environmental Health* (1974) 28:105–113.

Shambaugh, G., "Serous Otitis: Are Tubes the Answer?" *Pediatric Otology* (1983) 5(1):63–65.

Sharma, R., *Immunologic Considerations in Toxicology*, Vols. I and II (1981), CRC Press, Boca Raton, FL.

Shim, C., and Williams, M., "Effect of Odors in Asthma," *American Journal of Medicine* (1986) 80:18–22.

Shipley, M., "Transport of Molecules from Nose to Brain: Transneuronal Antigrade and Retrograde Labeling in the Rot Olfactory System by Wheat Germ Agglutirrin—Horseradish Peroxidane Applied to Nasal Epithelium," *Brain Research Bulletin* (1985) 15:129–142.

Shorter, R., "Idiopathic Inflammatory Bowel Disease: A Form of Food Allergy?" In: Brostoff, J., and Challacombe, S. (eds.) *Food Allergy and Intolerance* (1987), Bailliere Tindall, Philadelphia, 549–554.

Simon, G., et al., "Allergic to Life: Pychological Factors in Environmental Illness," *American Journal of Psychiatry* (1990) 147(7):901–906.

Skoldstam, L., "Effects of Diet on Rheumatoid Arthritis," *Internal Medicine for the Specialist* (1989) 10(5):128–137.

Sly, R.M., "Mortality from Asthma," *Journal of Allergy and Clinical Immunology* (1988) 82(5):705–717.

Snow, J., *Snow on Cholera* (1965; republished from 1936 original), Hoffner Publishing Company, New York, xxxvi.

Speizer, F., et al., "Palpitation Rates Associated with Fluorocarbon in a Hospital Setting," *New England Journal of Medicine* (1975) 292(12):624–626.

Spengler, J., Testimony Before the Ways and Means Committee, California State Legislature, February 22, 1988.

————, "Indoor Chemical Pollution," presentation given at the 46th Annual Meeting of the American College of Allergy and Immunology, Orlando, FL, November 15, 1989.

Spengler, J., and Sexton, K., "Indoor Air Pollution: A Public Health Perspective," *Science* (1983b) 221(4605):9–17.

Spengler, J., et al., "Nitrogen Dioxide inside and outside 137 Homes and Implications for Ambient Air Quality Standards and Health Effects Research," *Environmental Science and Technology* (1983a) 17(3):164–168.

Stankus, R., et al., "Cigarette Smoke–Sensitive Asthma: Challenge Studies," *Journal of Allergy and Clinical Immunology* (1988) 82(3, Pt 1):331–338.

Staudenmayer, H., presentation made at the Annual Meeting of the College of Allergy and Immunology, Orlando, FL, November 11, 1989.

Staudenmayer, H., and Camazini, M., "Sensing Type Personality, Projection and Universal 'Allergic' Reactivity," *Journal of Psychological Types* (1989).

Staudenmayer, H., and Selner, J., "Post-Traumatic Stress Syndrome (PTSS): Escape in the Environment," *Journal of Clinical Psychology* (1987) 43(1):156–157.

———, "Neuropsychophysiology during Relaxation in Generalized, Universal 'Allergic' Reactivity to the Environment: A Comparison Study," *Journal of Psychosomatic Research* (1990) 34(3):259–270.

Stein, M., et al., "The Hypothalamus and the Immune Response." In: Weiner, H., et al. (eds.), *Brain, Behavior and Bodily Disease* (1981), Raven Press, New York, 45–65.

Stokinger, H., "Ozone Toxicology," *Archives of Environmental Health* (1965) 10:719–731.

Strahilevitz, M., et al., "Air Pollutants and the Admission Rate of Psychiatric Patients," *American Journal of Psychiatry* (1979) 136(2):205–207.

Sullivan, T., Paper presented at the 45th Annual Meeting of the American Academy of Allergy and Immunology, San Antonio, Texas, February (1989).

Tabershaw, I., and Cooper, W., "Sequelae of Acute Organic Phosphate Poisoning," *Journal of Occupational Medicine* (1966) 8(1):5–20.

Taylor, G., and Harris, W., "Cardiac Toxicity of Aerosol Propellants," *Journal of the American Medical Association* (1970) 214(1):81–85.

Terr, A., "Environmental Illness: A Clinical Review of 50 Cases," *Archives of Internal Medicine* (1986) 146:145–149.

———, " 'Multiple Chemical Sensitivities': Immunological Critique of Clinical Ecology Theories and Practice." In: Cullen, M. (ed.) *Workers with Multiple Chemical Sensitivities* (1987), Hanley & Belfus, Philadelphia, 2(4):683–694.

———, "Clinical Ecology in the Workplace," *Journal of Occupational Medicine* (1989a) 31(3):257–261.

———, Remarks presented at the 45th Annual Meeting of the American Academy of Allergy and Immunology, San Antonio, Texas, February (1989b).

———, Personal communication, December 19, 1989 (1989c).

Thomson, G., *Report of the Ad Hoc Committee on Environmental Hypersensitivity Disorders* (1985) Ontario, Canada.

Thrasher, J., et al., "Evidence for Formaldehyde Antibodies and Altered Cellular Immunity in Subjects Exposed to Formaldehyde in Mobile Homes," *Archives of Environmental Health* (1987) 42(6):347–350.

———, "Building Related Illness and Antibodies to Albumin Conjugates of Formaldehyde, Toluene Diisocyanate, and Trimellitic Anhydride," *American Journal of Industrial Medicine* (1989) 15:187–195.

Tollerud, D., et al., "The Effects of Cigarette Smoking on T Cell Subsets," *American Review of Respiratory Diseases* (1989) 139(6):1446–1451.

Tretjak, Z., et al., "Occupational, Environmental, and Public Health in Semic: A Case Study of Polychlorinated Biphenyl (PCB) Pollution." In: Gunnerson, C. (ed.) *Post-Audits of Environmental Programs and Projects* (1989), American Society of Civil Engineers, 57–72.

Trounce, J., and Tanner, M., "Eosinophilic Gastroenteritis," *Archives of Diseases in Childhood* (1985) 60(12):1186–1188.

United States Congress, Office of Technology Assessment. *Neurotoxicity: Identifying and Controlling Poisons of the Nervous System*, OTA-BA-436, Washington, DC, April 1990.

United States Department of Labor, *An Interim Report to Congress on Occupational Diseases* (1980), Washington, DC

Urich, R., et al., "Does Suggestibility Modify Acute Reactions to Passive Cigarette Smoke?" *Environmental Research* (1988) 47:34–47.

Van Metre, T., Jr., and Adkinson, N., Jr., "Immunotherapy for Aeroallergen Disease." In: Middleton, E., Jr., et al. (eds.) *Allergy Principles and Practice*, Vol. II, 3d ed., (1988), C.V. Mosby Co., St. Louis, 1327–1343.

Van Sickle, G., et al., "Milk- and Soy Protein-Induced Enterocolitis: Evidence for Lymphocyte Sensitization to Specific Food Proteins," *Gastroenterology* (1985) 88(6):1915–1921.

Wachter, K., "Disturbed by Meta-Analysis?" *Science* (1988) 241:1407–1408.

Wallace, L., "Overview." In: Gammage, R., and Kaye, S. (eds.) *Indoor Air and Human Health* (1985), Lewis Publishers, Chelsea, MI, 331–333.

————, "The TEAM Study: Personal Exposures to Toxic Substances in Air, Drinking Water, and Breath of 400 Residents of New Jersey, North Carolina, and North Dakota," *Environmental Research* (1987) 43:290–307.

Wallace, L., et al., "Organic Chemicals in Indoor Air: A Review of Human Exposure Studies and Indoor Air Quality Studies." In: Gammage, R., and Kaye, S. (eds.) *Indoor Air and Human Health* (1985), Lewis Publishers, Chelsea, MI, 361–378.

Walsh, T., and Emerich, D., "The Hippocampus as a Common Target of Neurotoxic Agents," *Toxicology* (1988)49:137–140.

Wasner, C., et al., "The Use of Unproven Remedies," *Scientific American* (1980) 23(1):759–760.

Winkelmann, R., "Food Sensitivity and Urticaria or Vasculitis." In: Brostoff, J., and Challacombe, S. (eds.) *Food Allergy and Intolerance* (1987), Bailliere Tindall, Philadelphia, 602–617.

Wojtulewski, J., "Joints and Connective Tissue." In: Brostoff, J., and Challacombe, S. (eds.) *Food Allergy and Intolerance* (1987), Bailliere Tindall, Philadelphia, 723–736.

Wolff, M., et al., "Equilibrium of Polybrominated Biphenyl (PBB) Residues in Serum and Fat of Michigan Residents," *Bulletin of Environmental Contamination and Toxicology* (1979) 21(6):775–781.

————, "Human Tissue Burdens of Halogenated Aromatic Chemicals in Michigan," *Journal of the American Medical Association* (1982) 247(15):2112–2116.

Wraith, D., "Asthma." In: Brostoff, J., and Challacombe, S. (eds.) *Food Allergy and Intolerance* (1987), Bailliere Tindall, Philadelphia, 486–497.

Yu, D., et al., "Peripheral Blood Ia-Positive T cells," *Journal of Experimental Medicine* (1980) 151:91–100.

Zamm, A., and Gannon, R., *Why Your House May Endanger Your Health* (1980), Simon and Schuster, New York.

Ziem, G., Personal communication, November 8, 1989.

Index

Page numbers in *italics* refer to figures; page numbers in **boldface** refer to tables.